DILEMMA

A Nurse's Guide for Making Ethical Decisions

Judith Allen Shelly

InterVarsity Press
Downers Grove
Illinois 60515

InterVarsity Press is the book-publishing division of Inter-Varsity Christian Fellowship, a student movement active on campus at hundreds of universities, colleges and schools of nursing. For information about local and regional activities, write IVCF, 233 Langdon St., Madison, WI 53703.

Distributed in Canada through InterVarsity Press, 1875 Leslie St., Unit 10, Don Mills, Ontario M3B 2M5, Canada.

Biblical quotations are from the Revised Standard Version of the Bible, copyrighted 1946, 1952, © 1971, 1973, and are used by permission. The two opening letters of the Preface are used by permission from Lynne Cole and Sister Corrine.

Acknowledgments:
The ANA "Code for Nurses" is reprinted with permission from Code for Nurses with Interpretive Statements © American Nurses' Association, 1976.

The ICN "Code for Nurses" is reprinted with permission from Barbara L. Tate, The Nurse's Dilemma, Ethical Considerations in Nursing Practice © 1977 by the International Council of Nurses, Geneva, Switzerland.

"Patient's Bill of Rights" is reprinted with the permission of the American Hospital Association, © 1975.

"Living Will" is reprinted with permission from Concern for Dying, 250 West 57th Street, New York, New York 10019.

"Christian Affirmation of Life" is reprinted with permission of The Catholic Health Association. Copies are available from the Publications Department, CHA, 1438 S. Grand Blvd., St. Louis, MO 63104.

"Instructions for My Care in the Event of Terminal Illness" is reprinted with permission of the American Protestant Hospital Association, 1701 E. Woodfield Road, Schaumburg, IL 60195.

ISBN 0-87784-666-9

Printed in the United States of America

Library of Congress Cataloging in Publication Data
Shelly, Judith Allen.
    Dilemma: a nurse's guide for making ethical decisions.

    Bibliography: p.
    1. Nursing ethics.   2. Christian ethics.
3. Medicine and Christianity.   I. Title.
[DNLM: 1. Decision making.   2. Ethics, Nursing.
WY85 S545d]
RT85.S47   174'.2   80-7788
ISBN 0-87784-666-9

17	16	15	14	13	12	11	10	9	8	7	6	5	4	3	2	1
94	93	92	91	90	89	88	87	86	85	84	83	82	81	80		

Preface

Reflections: An Open Letter to God
Re: The Basis for Ethics—Especially Mine

From: Lynne, a Nurse
To: God in Heaven
Please Forward to Sister Corrine

Good Morning, Lord,

It's me—Lynne—I need to talk with you. I surely am glad You're always available. It's great to know that I have a Lord who never slumbers nor sleeps (Ps. 121:4). Sometimes I need to talk to You even when I should be sleeping.

Anyway, Lord, what I wanted to talk to you about this morning is this class I'm taking at the hospital—Ethical Dilemmas in Health Care—Wow! there certainly are plenty of those! Just this week I confronted a doctor about not returning phone calls—I shocked myself!—but those two old ladies were really sick and fading fast. (One died later that day.) The doctor sent me a letter later through the nursing office. Oh dear! Lord, I make no apologies! I *know* I did the right thing.

I seem to be getting sidetracked, but it's all related to what I want to talk with You about—this ethics class. Sister Corrine is delightful and makes us feel comfortable and not threatened about expressing ourselves— that's important to me—especially in an area as personal as *my* ethics.

A while back, Lord, it was kind of scary, especially afterwards. I refused to post-date a consent for a pacemaker. A doctor actually asked me to do that—Imagine! and he is (or was) a respected cardiologist. I guess that basically I'm a "truth-teller"—now that can get you in hot water in a hurry! I really do try to be very careful about *how* I say things though.

I've thought a lot about where I am ethically since returning to nursing, and this class has certainly made me glad that I have a firm foundation to operate from. Sometimes when the pressure is on and I'm tempted to question whether it's worth it, You're always there to confirm over and over again that it is indeed worth it. Thanks.

Sometimes I feel sad that for twenty-five years I was unaware of the firm base You provide. Thank You, though, for giving me parents who provided an *unbending* moral and ethical structure—which, I have to admit (regrettably), I resisted at times.

Since I committed my life to You over twenty years ago now the "foundation for my house" has been firm—I'm grateful. Luke made some interesting comparisons for us to enjoy. I like the one about the houses—the one stood unshaken because it was built on a deep rock foundation, but the other collapsed in ruin since it had no foundation. Luke says the firm foundation is Your Word and that my actions are the house (Luke 6:47-49). Wow! That's really something—that seems to place a lot of responsibility on me for right actions, Lord. Am I ever glad that you said, "I will never desert . . . nor . . . forsake you" (Hebrews 13:5).

It gets sticky at work sometimes and I do want to do what is right and fair. I must admit that I do get quite incensed when my sense of fairness is violated. I know I need to watch my "incensed" level—thanks for helping me with that.

Lord, You know that I really enjoy Paul's letters. Timothy must have been delighted when those two letters arrived. I've been reading them lately. (It's fun to read other people's mail.) A few things Paul said are again really important to me—especially now that I'm taking this class—and now that I must re-evaluate my own ethical base. May I reiterate?

"Discipline yourself for the purpose of godliness (1 Timothy 4:7). . . . In speech, conduct, love, faith and purity, show yourself an example of those who believe (4:12). . . . [Store] up . . . the good treasure of a good foundation for the future . . . [to] take hold of that which is life indeed" (6:19).

"Difficult times will come (2 Timothy 3:1) ... [with people] always learning and never able to come to the knowledge of the truth (3:7). ... Continue in the things you have learned and become convinced of, knowing from whom you have learned them [You, Lord, and Your] ... sacred writings ... inspired by God ... [so that I] ... may be adequate, equipped for every good work" (3:14-17). What a relief to have my foundation (my ethical base) reaffirmed. Thank you, Lord.

Oh my! I've gone on and on! How well You know that I seldom write letters, and then they are brief! I'm supposed to write a paper for this class. Oh dear! I'll never get these thoughts condensed and organized into a formal two page paper—or even an informal one. Perhaps Sister Corrine won't mind just reading Your letter. Please pass it on to her.

Thanks for listening,
Lynne, a nurse on Earth

Dear Lynne,

Thank you for your very thoughtful and sensitive letter. I felt privileged to read it! You have been gifted and blessed with a "firm foundation" —a solid grounding for your values. Your personal belief in the Lord's love for you and for others and the conviction that being His friend makes certain demands on us gives you the strength to take a difficult stand. (One thing I got from reading your letter is that I'd feel more comfortable being a patient on a floor where you worked!)

You clearly recognize that the issues are difficult, and that it is risky to challenge physicians, or others whom you feel are violating some ethical principle. Yet, you are willing to search your own conscience and stick your neck out if you see the need. Actually, this love affair you have with the Lord almost requires that of you. He clearly wants to reach others through you. My personal thanks to you for accepting that responsibility. It won't always be easy or free of tension—in fact, almost never, as you know! But you have a courage which is "not of this world."

Thanks also for your affirmation of me. It meant a lot!

Sister Corrine

Do Lynne's dilemmas sound familiar? From the very first time you set foot in a hospital as a nursing student you probably began to face ethical dilemmas. Making ethical decisions probably did not come easy then, nor has it likely become any easier since. None of us like to make ethical decisions, especially those that may lead us into confrontation with others. Yet the nature of our profession requires us constantly to make moral and ethical judgments.

Moral values and ethical conduct spring from inner convictions and a personal philosophy of life. For the Christian the basis for making ethical decisions comes from a relationship with Jesus Christ. As Sister Corrine said to Lynne, "You are willing to search your own conscience and stick your neck out if you see the need. Actually, this love affair you have with the Lord almost requires that of you."

Though cast headfirst into making ethical decisions by the nature of nursing and the demands of faith, few of us feel adequate for the task. My experience suggests that even more than help with *what* to think about ethics, we need help with *how* to think about ethics. This book is designed to fill that need. It is not an exposition of philosophical ethics or an explanation of various ethical positions, but rather a guidebook to help nurses learn how to think through the wide variety of ethical dilemmas which commonly arise in nursing practice.

Part one lays a foundation by establishing a framework for making ethical decisions. The first two chapters examine the important relationship between ethics and nursing practice. Chapters three through eight introduce a comprehensive process for making ethical decisions which is carefully illustrated from clinical experiences.

Part two takes you a step further. First, a preliminary study helps you to think through your own philosophy of nursing. Then a series of eight clinical case studies enables you to apply the decision-making process of Part one to concrete situations. A set of guidelines for discussion groups follows, which, if used, will stimulate further growth. Each study is demanding but will provide solid preparation for making ethical decisions in the real world of nursing.

Part One
A Process for Making Ethical Decisions

1
Ethics:
What? Why?

He has showed you, O man, what is good;
   and what does the LORD require of you
but to do justice, and to love kindness,
   and to walk humbly with your God?
Micah 6:8

Why can't they just let mother die a natural death?" Margaret sobbed to the chaplain as personnel rushed into her mother's hospital room to begin resuscitation efforts for the second time in a week. Her mother, Mary O'Brian, had undergone surgery for carcinoma of the colon earlier in the week and had had a cardiac arrest on the operating table. Margaret saw the arrest as God's way of taking her mother painlessly rather than subjecting her to the agonies of cancer. She was angry that the surgeon had thwarted "God's plan."

As the weeks wore on Mrs. O'Brian suffered five more cardiac arrests before she finally died. During that time Margaret and several nurses had pleaded with the attending physician for a "no code" status for Mrs. O'Brian. He refused. Discussion at the nurses' station grew heated as the number of successful resuscitations increased.

"It's not fair. Why do we keep torturing this poor lady? . . . So she can get well to go home and die of cancer?"

"But her cancer hasn't metasticized. All the nodes were clean. She could still lead a normal life."

"Yes, but it's tearing her family apart. I don't see how they can stand it. Each time she arrests they start the grief process all over again. I wonder how much longer they can take it."

"I'm beginning to agree with her daughter. We're sitting here playing God. Mama dies, so we push the magic God-stopper button and bring her back to life again."

"Well, a person isn't dead until their brain stops functioning, and I believe that God gives us the responsibility to preserve life as long as we can."

"Maybe you're right, but I don't know how much longer I can take it." ∎

Nurses face ethical dilemmas every day. The very nature of nursing brings us into constant contact with conflicting values in an atmosphere of tension and immediacy. In each situation the decisions we make, or refuse to make, often have far-reaching ramifications. As the nursing profession assumes more and more independence and responsibility, the need for ethical decision making increases. We will be held accountable for the decisions we make, both morally and legally.

If you were one of the nurses caring for Mrs. O'Brian what would you do? Would you conscientiously resuscitate her after each arrest and feel right in doing so? Would you keep on calling "codes" but also plead with the physician to stop them? Would you take your time getting to the phone to call a "code" the next time she arrested, hoping this time she would become sufficiently anoxic to die? What kind of care would you give Mrs. O'Brian in the meantime? How would you support her family? How would you communicate your ethical stance to other nursing personnel?

Ethical decision making is a complicated process. It is an outgrowth of personal beliefs and values, and of a philosophy of life and nursing. It is also influenced by culture and emotions. But before examining the decision-making process, perhaps we should back up. Just what is ethics?

What Is Ethics?

Abortion and euthanasia always come to the forefront whenever nursing ethics is discussed. Any time matters of life and death arise where a measure of human control is involved, an ethical dilemma is created. But ethics covers a broader scope than the dramatic crisis situations of euthanasia and abortion. Ethics is the science of morals. It attempts to answer the questions of what is right and wrong, good and bad, and of how to achieve the good. At the individual level ethics is the conscious and systematic choice of moral values by which a person governs his or her conduct.

Although many of us have been taught to shun making value judgments, in fact, to consider making value judgments the ultimate sin in nursing practice, the truth is that no nurse can avoid making value judgments. The issue is whether our moral choices will be made consciously and willfully or blindly and haphazardly.

The goal of ethics is to ensure that the right and the good prevail. When the choice between good and evil is clear, decisions are easy. When an accident victim is brought into the emergency room, no difficulty arises in deciding whether or not to begin treatment. If after admission, however, the patient suffers a cardiac arrest from which he or she is resuscitated but never regains consciousness, then an ethical dilemma may develop. Suppose another patient with a better prognosis for recovery arrives, requiring the bed and respirator of the first patient. To whom should the respirator be given and to whom should it be denied? The decision is no longer simple. Now there is a choice between two goods (giving adequate treatment to either patient) or two corresponding evils (denying adequate treatment to the other patient). Here the need for clear, principled thinking, as opposed to spur-of-the-moment, haphazard choosing, is evident.

To say, as I have, that there should be no question about whether to initiate the treatment of an accident victim in the emergency room assumes that a common ethic, based on a common set of values, already exists. In general, we readily assume the value of human life, but we do not have to look far to find that such value is not and has not been universally assumed. In another culture, or another period of history, such a person might have been left to die or used for experimentation. For example, Patrick Romanell, professor of philosophy at the University of Texas, El Paso, notes that health care in classical Greece, when judged by contemporary standards, left much to be desired. Weak infants were destroyed, and there was never any organized system of care for cripples or the blind: "In short, the classical Greek patient was burdened with the stigma of 'inferiority,' from which he 'was freed by Christianity.' . . . Classical Greek ethics and Christian ethics are not the same in general outlook, and their different conceptions of the good life show up in matters of health as elsewhere."[1]

In the United States we have been blessed with a system of ethics in nursing which stems from a Judeo-Christian heritage. It is a system which assumes the sanctity of human life and which regards compassion and caring for the sick as duties of society. But these values can quickly erode even in a so-called Christian nation as Nazi Germany so readily reminds us. The atrocities committed there show us how fragile and dynamic a society's basis for ethical decision making really is.

Why Study Ethics?

According to nursing ethicist Myra E. Levine, "We are a generation frightened by our ability to influence decisions relating to life and death yet, at the same time, unable to fix guidelines for compassion and justice."[2] In this context ethics has become an area of increasing concern among nurses. What once seemed obvious and easy to decide has now become confusing. Where once nurses functioned from a common set of values encapsulated in the Nightingale Pledge, we are now confronted with a variety of conflicting values.

We live in a pluralistic society made up of many faith and belief systems. In our diversity can we still arrive at common values in health care? If not, then who decides what is best for a patient? If the patient is the one to decide, then how is a nurse to function when the patient demands services which conflict with the nurse's values? For example, what does a nurse do if a patient demands a fatal dose of morphine?

We are unsure about the nature of our relationships to patients, physicians or other health-care professionals. We are obsessed with rights and question the validity of responsibilities. We live in the midst of sensual society; feelings are one of the only absolutes we accept. We have been convinced that facts can prove anything and that laws are made to be broken. As Diane Uustal, writing in the *Sigma Theta Tau/ Image*, states, "Ideally, our feelings and decisions are based on our values, but sometimes we are unclear about what it is we value. Every day, as professional nurses, each of us meets situations which call for careful analysis, decision making, affirmative action, and accountability."[3] If we do not know what we value, or why we value certain concepts, beliefs, attitudes and behaviors, then we cannot make responsible ethical decisions. Thus our need to study ethics and the process of ethical decision making becomes evident.

"Oh, but I'm a Christian!" you may respond. "I know what I believe." Yet, how often do we Christians fail to consider the implications of our doctrinal beliefs for everyday decision making?

Christians live in the same world as everybody else. We are influenced by the trends, fads and concerns of the world around us. Our attitudes and ideas are shaped by the same schools, newspapers, television programs and insitutional policies as our neighbors'. Often, when the time for ethical decisions arises, we are just as confused as those who do not share our beliefs. When one Christian nurse was asked how she handled making ethical decisions, she spoke for many, "I try not to think about them."

Uustal, in the same periodical article, asks, "Are you aware that the clearer we are about what we value, the more able we are to choose and initiate a response which is consistent with what we say we believe?"[4] The purpose of studying ethics is to prepare ourselves to behave ethically when faced with a dilemma, to learn to function consistently with what we believe.

Consider some of the opinions you now hold. Do you believe that a person has the right to end his own life if he wants to? Do you feel nurses have the right to strike? Do you think that you should have the right to refuse to care for abortion patients? Do you think health-care agencies should pay for the further education of nurses they employ? Do you think peer review is a good thing?

What influences most affect your answers to these questions and others like them? Your religious unbringing? Your study of Scripture? Your nursing education? Your hospital experience? A study of ethics will help you to determine what you believe, why you believe it and how to act on it.

Put simply, Christian ethics is faith in action. It involves getting to know God and attempting to do his will in everyday situations. Because Christian ethics assumes Scripture as a starting point for ethical decision making, it requires searching the Scriptures prayerfully and applying them to daily life. As in other areas of the Christian life this is one in which we can gain from the guidance, support and encouragement of other Christians.

We live in a time and a society where values are rapidly changing. Often the changes are subtle, and we are swept along with the apparent logic of the trends. As Christians we need to have a firm grasp of biblical content and a clear understanding of how to apply it to ethical decision making. We need to be aware of our ethical responsibilities as nurses and to be able to recognize the issues at stake in the ethical dilemmas that confront us. We need to know how to find God's will in these dilemmas and how to take action based on our understanding of it. The prophet Micah gave us some useful guidelines:

He has showed you, O man, what is good;
and what does the LORD require of you
but to do justice, and to love kindness,
and to walk humbly with your God? (Micah 6:8)

Justice, kindness and a humble walk with God—timeless advice for ethical behavior in a technical environment with shifting values. Let us explore together that advice and its implications for nursing.

2
Ethics and Nursing

I solemnly pledge myself *before God*
and in the presence of this assembly
to pass my life in purity and to practice
my profession faithfully. I will
abstain from whatever is deleterious
and mischievous, and will not
take or knowingly administer any harmful drug. I will do all in my power
to maintain and elevate the standard
of my profession, and will hold
in confidence all personal matters
committed to my keeping and all
family affairs coming to my knowledge
in the practice of my calling. With
loyalty will I endeavor to aid
the physician in his work, and devote
myself to the welfare of those
committed to my care.
The Florence Nightingale Pledge

What is your philosophy of nursing? What do you think constitutes good nursing practice? What qualities do you feel a nurse should possess? If you are answering these questions as you read, you are beginning to think about ethics in nursing. Surprised? You thought nursing ethics dealt with profound subjects of life and death importance? Well, it may, but until we put it into the context of nursing practice and personal responsibility, we are not talking *nursing* ethics.

For years nurses have discussed ethics in the third person, as spectators rather than participants. Major topics like abortion, euthanasia, genetic engineering and transplant surgery were placed under the heading of "medical ethics," which absolved us of any real responsibility. The assumption was that physicians alone made these ethical decisions. Nurses merely carried out doctors' decisions, unless the orders seemed outright harmful or dangerous. Then, and only then, did nurses refuse to follow physicians' orders.

In a Hastings Center Report on ethical issues in nursing practice, ethicist Andrew Jameton states, "Most bioethics teaching in nursing has consisted in simply extending the teaching of standard medical ethics issues to a new audience—nurses. This is a mistake. The practice of nursing gives rise to a variety of ethical problems either unique to the profession or significantly modified by it."[1] In Jameton's view these problems arise from (1) a conflict of roles, (2) a unique concept of health care as a "unified science" and (3) the need to work within a team of professionals, each with their own frames of reference, cultural baggage and historical struggles for recognition and influence. Let's examine these sources of problems.

Role Conflict

Nurses have a unique relationship with patients. We probably spend more time with patients than any other member of the health team. We are usually more available in times of crisis. We often fulfill the role of coordinator of patient services and function as a liaison between the patient and other health professionals. Because of this unique relationship we become advocates for the patient in many ethical dilemmas. For instance, a physician who orders a lethal dose of morphine may be questioned by a nurse. A dietary department that does not want to bring a late tray for a patient who was in X ray during lunch must reckon with a nurse. A nurse who gives poor or unsafe care may be reviewed by both peers and supervisors.

But nurses are not only responsible to the patients in their care, they are also responsible to hospital administrators, to physicians writing orders and to God. These differing roles then give rise to ethical problems unique to nurses. Patients need compassionate, skilled nursing care. Hospital administrators need good public relations and a realistic budget. Physicians expect nurses to carry out plans of medical treatment. But often the hospital's tight budget works against compassionate care because it results in understaffing. The need for good public relations may prevent honest disclosure of serious errors, such as those reported not long ago in several Philadelphia area operating rooms, where oxygen and nitrous oxide gas lines were reversed, resulting in a number of deaths.

At times the physicians' orders may be obviously harmful to the patient, but they may refuse to change them, forcing nurses to decide whether to follow them or, perhaps, to lose their jobs. In other cases patients, hospitals and physicians may be in agreement with their demands upon nurses, but those demands may be in conflict with nurses' personal beliefs and values. For instance, in a case involving Siamese twins joined at the chest, it was known that one twin would die as a result of surgery to separate them. As a result several nurses refused to participate in the operation.[2]

Health Care as a Unified Science

Nurses usually view patients as whole persons. Although most physicians would agree in principle, nurses frequently become frustrated when patients are treated as assemblies of organs by specialists dealing with only one set of organs. What should a nurse do when a brittle diabetic is being prepared for major surgery while his diabetes is being ignored or grossly mismanaged by the surgeon? Or what about a dying patient who seems to have a deep need to discuss his death with family and nursing personnel but is kept so sedated that he cannot think or talk clearly? Or what is the responsibility of a nurse in a situation like this? A patient is seen by a cardiologist on consultation and told she has a heart murmur. Then the patient, seeing the attending physician who had ordered the consultation, asks him what the implications of her heart murmur are. His only response is, "I wish cardiologists were born mute."

Nurses as Team Members

Nurses usually think of themselves as part of a team. The team consists of other nurses, physicians, physical therapists, laboratory technologists, x-ray technicians and other paramedical professionals and nonprofessionals. Because of this multidisciplinary involvement in patient care, nursing ethics cannot take place in isolation from other team members. Traditionally the physician has been "the one who decides," but that role is being challenged, and rightly so, for today's ethical decisions are too big for any one person to assume total responsibility.

The uniqueness of nursing ethics is found in the uniqueness of nursing. It is the quest for justice and mercy within our realm of responsibility and influence as nurses. For the Christian nurse, the standards for justice and mercy will be found in God's will as it is expressed in his Word and understood by his people.

Leah Curtin, acting director of the National Center for Nursing Ethics, provides an example of nursing ethics by considering the possible role of nursing in the euthanasia question. She points out that many of the individuals at risk are within the concern of nursing: "Those individuals who are chronically ill, dying, aged or seriously handicapped frequently seem to offer little challenge to medicine, i.e. 'the art of curing,' but they offer a tremendous challenge to nursing, i.e. 'the art of caring.' The contrast between nursing and medicine could not be clearer."[3] She suggests that nurses will be involved on three levels: (1) on an individual level, with individual patients, (2) on a decision-making level, interacting with physicians, family members and ethicists, and (3) on a societal level, influencing legislation and social policies. She concludes, "The role of the nurse and nursing in the multi-faceted 'euthanasia' controversy may well be, but is not limited to, providing the alternatives to what may appear to be an 'either/or' situation."[4]

Nursing is also involved with all the mundane routines of health care as well as the dramatic life and death crises; therefore, nursing ethics also includes the everyday decisions about use of time, truth-telling, fairness in assignments, accurate record keeping and provision of consistent quality nursing care.

Ethics in a Growing Profession

A popular text on nursing ethics written over fifty years ago gives four guiding principles on the ethical duties of nursing students. Every nursing student should:

[1] meekly accept, as right and necessary, much that she cannot understand. . . .

[2] try to see every situation from the viewpoint of those in authority. . . .

[3] analyze her own motives and be sure that they are pure and unselfish. . . .

[4] pay careful attention to what is said by those placed in authority over the school.[5]

Today most of us would consider it downright dangerous to accept anything as "right and necessary" if we did not understand it. The motives and actions of "those in authority" are regularly questioned and challenged. In some cases an impartial mediator must be brought in to communicate the viewpoints of those in authority to staff nurses, and of staff nurses to those in authority. Many nurses consider "pure and unselfish" motives to be detrimental for nurses when it comes to achieving an increase in salary and benefits. Students are no longer forced to conform to an authoritarian system but are encouraged to think for themselves.

In general, the changes in nursing and nurses have been positive steps of growth. We are better educated, more independent, more responsible and creatively working toward more thorough and comprehensive health care for a wider range of patients. But growth is always painful.

Nursing ethics was much simpler when all a nurse had to do was to follow the rules and the doctor's orders. As we expand our realm of responsibility and influence we also enlarge the scope of our ethical decision making and the need to be well informed so that responsible decisions can be made. Nursing ethics must keep pace with nursing practice in order to be relevant. We must keep up to date on the issues at stake, maintaining competence in our fields and considering each aspect of our professional practice in the light of our personal beliefs.

As nursing has changed, so have various codes of nursing. The American Nurses' Association Code for Nurses, the International Council of Nurses Code for Nurses and the American Hospital Association Patient's Bill of Rights are all codes with which we should be familiar (see appendix for copies of each). These codes are based on basic common beliefs about human rights and needs. While the codes are not legally binding, they provide guidelines for acceptable professional behavior.

Sometimes ethical dilemmas arise when personal beliefs and values conflict with commonly accepted professional standards. For instance, the ANA Code for Nurses states: "The nurse, acting through the professional organization, participates in establishing and maintaining conditions of employment conducive to high-quality nursing care." On the surface this sounds like an admirable standard, but some nurses have found that following it may mean walking a picket line while patients receive minimal care. You may not agree, but my beliefs and values would keep me from participating in such a strike.

Nursing ethics is a new field, yet an old concern for nurses. What has been taught about nursing ethics in schools of nursing has been scant and varied.[6] In a pluralistic society it is difficult, if not impossible, to determine a common basis for moral behavior, but nurses are grasping for guidelines and leadership in ethical decision making. If you want your voice to be heard when ethical guidelines are established, now is the time to develop your philosophy of nursing, based on what you believe about God, humanity and the world around you. Future codes of nursing, legislation and curriculum offerings on nursing ethics will be shaped by those who speak out most loudly and clearly during this time of growth and transition.

3
Assuming Ethical Responsibility

To be a nurse requires the willing
assumption of ethical responsibility in
every dimension of practice.
Myra E. Levine

Ethical decision making, to be responsible, must be systematic. You probably would not consider giving nursing care to a patient without a nursing care plan, but how often have you made ethical decisions with minimal assessment of the apparent problem?

An ethical dilemma, by its very nature, involves tension and conflict. It is extremely difficult to remain objective in the midst of such situations. Most of us fall back on intuition and make decisions based on our feelings of the moment. We are often not even aware of the complex issues involved.

While most Christians come into nursing with a strong sense of right and wrong and a basic working knowledge of the Bible, few have examined how those beliefs apply in situations where they apparently conflict or appear inapplicable.

Our primary concern as Christians in an ethical dilemma is to discern God's will, yet in the flurry and commotion of the situation we may find it difficult to hear God's voice. Just as Elijah, in 1 Kings 19, could not find God in the wind or the earthquake or the fire, we may also have to temporarily withdraw from the pressures of the immediate situation to hear God speaking in a "still small voice." When Elijah finally heard God's voice, God said, "What are you doing here, Elijah?" (v. 13). Elijah explained, "I have been very jealous for the LORD, the God of hosts; for the people of Israel have forsaken thy covenant, thrown down thy altars, and slain thy prophets with the sword; and I, even I only, am left; and they seek my life, to take it away" (v. 14). The Lord then sent him back into the battle with a clear set of directions.

All too often we begin to think like Elijah. We see ourselves as God's lone defender in a secular world and plunge into a situation proclaiming God's will without consulting him first. Instead, we need to draw back and systematically evaluate each ethical dilemma confronting us, all the while listening to that "still small voice" of God. In doing so, we may discover that God's directions will frequently differ from our initial visceral reactions. Elijah, following his intuition, ended up about 400 miles in the opposite direction from where God wanted him. While claiming to be the Lord's lone defender, he was camped out in a cave on the side of Mt. Horeb (Mt. Sinai), taking refuge in a safe place where the law of God had been proclaimed. In the meantime, there were 7,000 others left in Israel who were faithful to God and desperate for leadership.

Yet, we shouldn't come down too hard on poor old Elijah. How often have you heard Christians—yourself?—say, "If nurses in our hospital unionize, I'm leaving!" or "If doctors in our hospital perform abortions, I'm going somewhere else!"? In the rush to get away we can miss seeing alternatives and leave other Christians in the situation without support or leadership, while we take refuge in a safe "Christian" environment. The Christian's task in making a systematic study of ethical dilemmas is to learn how to live *in* the world without being *of* it (Jn. 17:15-19).

What we need to learn is how to be the "salt of the earth" and the "light of the world" that Jesus appointed us to be in Matthew 5:13-16. Salt both adds flavor and preserves. By being salt we can help people see God's meaning and purpose in life, and preserve his moral standards in the world. As lights of the world we may reveal the selfish motives and disastrous consequences of violating God's law, as well as present the redemption Jesus Christ offers in the midst of seemingly impossible situations. In order to do that we need to be adequately informed about all aspects of the ethical dilemmas which surround us. We must be praying, thinking, studying the Scriptures, reading, talking, listening and leaning on God all the way.

Looking at the Process

The first step in ethical decision making is assessment. Just as you would assess your patient before making a nursing intervention, you can assess an ethical dilemma. Observing, investigating and interpreting are important aspects of assessment. We need to look specifically at how to clarify the personal context of a dilemma—identifying emotional responses, exploring personal biases, examining cultural values and opening interpersonal communications. After gaining a more objective perspective, we can begin to define the problem by determining who is involved, what issues are at stake and what further information is necessary to make an informed decision.

The next step in our dilemma "care plan" is planning. At this point we can begin to propose alternatives—first brainstorming about every conceivable option, then considering the feasibility and effects of each alternative. There is always more than one alternative in a dilemma, and usually more than two or three. The purpose of systematic planning at this stage is to avoid becoming locked into a frantic "either/or" situation. We can then begin to interpret the meaning of the data collected and evaluate alternatives by looking at Scripture and reading the works of ethicists, theologians and other informed Christians, as well as talking and praying with others in the Christian community. Just as a nursing care plan is useless unless it leads to action, the planning stage in making an ethical decision is not complete until we have determined a workable plan of action and communicated it to everyone involved.

In nursing ethics we do not have the luxury of sitting back in an ivory tower, speculating on purely hypothetical situations. We are surrounded by a plethora of real life dilemmas. A *plan* of action is not enough. We not only want to *know* God's will, but to *do* it as well. Intervention is our primary goal. Responsible, effective intervention which reflects God's character and communicates his concern for all persons involved in the situation should be the outcome of our approach to ethical decision making.

To be helpful a systematic process for making ethical decisions should free us to make informed, responsible decisions. The decision-making process which is described and illustrated in the following chapters is not a lockstep procedure which must be followed rigidly. It is a dynamic process. Each point in the outline will define and clarify aspects of the dilemma, which will prepare you to move on to the next step; but you may also find that one step will lead you to rethink an earlier one. For example, evaluating alternatives may suggest new alternatives, or reading legal aspects may reveal totally new issues involved, or listening to what other Christians say may cause you to re-examine the Scriptures. The purpose of following a systematic method in decision making is to have a comprehensive strategy that will prevent your missing important points along the way. It helps you to cut through the quagmire of the situation and keep your ears and heart open to the "still small voice" of God.

The situations that follow are not hypothetical. They really happened. They are not pure, one-issue dilemmas, but are complicated by the humanity of each person involved. Fears, frustrations and interpersonal communication problems color each situation as much as moral values and personal beliefs. In other words, they represent the real world of nursing ethics. I hope that after studying them you will be not only informed, but also encouraged. Being embroiled in an ethical dilemma can be a frightening and lonely experience. The temptation is always there to think, like Elijah, that "I, even I only, am left." In working through these case studies you can take heart that you are not alone. Others have gone before, have felt the pain, have struggled with the frustrations; and still others remain in the situation with you, willing to support you as you seek to do God's will.

4
Clarifying the Personal Context

Step I. Clarify the Personal Context
A. Identify emotional responses
B. Explore personal biases
C. Examine cultural values
D. Open interpersonal communications

A sea of muddy water often clouds the ethical dilemmas which nurses face. Emotional responses, personal biases, cultural values and poor interpersonal communications can prevent the clear recognition of an ethical dilemma, or can appear to create a dilemma which does not really exist. If a moral problem is recognized, these same factors can interfere with a nurse's ability to clearly define and analyze the situation at hand.

Emotions color many of our beliefs, attitudes and actions. Often our own defense mechanisms keep us from recognizing how much emotional responses affect our nursing practice. A study conducted in a large general hospital determined that nurses usually hurried to answer the calls of patients who were far from death, but responded more slowly to the calls of patients near death. When the nurses were confronted with the results of the study, they vigorously denied the facts.[1] Fear of death created a moral problem, for dying patients received care inferior to that given healthier patients.

Emotions sway our assessment of ethical dilemmas. I vividly remember an incident early in my nursing career. A young mother who had severely battered her first child became pregnant. I had cared for her first child each time he was beaten, thrown down the stairs, burned or generally abused. As a newborn he had been a soft, cuddly baby who easily snuggled into my arms. At age two he was tense and frightened and moved away from anyone who came near him. Finally he was placed in a foster home. Now that his mother was pregnant again all I could think about was how I wished she could have an abortion (it was illegal at the time). I was unable to see the mother's needs or to consider the moral implications of abortion. All I could envision was another baby with broken bones, bruises and burns; and all I could feel was anger toward the mother.

Personal biases are another subtle influence in our ethical decision making. It is much easier to give good care to a patient you like and approve of than to one who has violated your personal standards. One evening when receiving the change of shift report, I began to respond to a patient's call light. The nurse reporting off replied, "Oh, that's just that whiny kid in isolation. He got hepatitis from using dirty needles to shoot up with drugs. Serves him right!" She turned his light off at the desk without checking to see what he wanted, "You've got to be firm with kids like this, they're used to having their own way all the time." I am sure that this nurse thought that what she had done was right. She was unaware that by so doing she had denied the patient his right to be heard.

Sometimes our overt behavior toward patients may not be affected as much as our attitudes about them, but by those attitudes we may influence other personnel. For instance, a nurse admitted a male patient who was scheduled for a rhinoplasty. He explained to her that this was the first stage in a series of operations which would be concluded with a sex-change operation. She came out of his room waving his clothing list and giggling, "You wouldn't believe what this guy brought with him! A lacy nightie for each day he's expecting to be here!" Her response set a precedent, and the patient became the joke of the unit, each nurse trying to outdo the others with stories of what the patient had done. He received good physical care, but because he was not taken seriously as a person he received little emotional support.

Cultural values are closely tied to our emotions and personal biases, but their effects are broader. Their influence is often difficult to recognize because they are so widely accepted that they become our standards of right and wrong. Paul Langham states, "When nurses are called upon to make moral decisions, they make them simply on the basis of 'moral intuitions,' grounded in uncritically accepted religious, societal, and legal mores. . . . Unfortunately, our moral intuitions are rarely subjected to systematic analysis and frequently even turn out to be mutually incompatible."[2]

Such an incompatibility is becoming evident now in our society with the abortion issue. Until recently the sanctity of individual human life was respected from conception to death. Abortion was considered both illegal and immoral. Now abortion is legal, and many people consider it not only moral, but commendable. For example, Rosalee Yeaworth writes in the *American Journal of Nursing,* "If the $900,000 spared for each averted case of severe retardation could be diverted to providing good health care to all, then the grounds for social concern in relation to amniocentesis and abortion are obvious."[3] She goes on to suggest that some people feel society should require amniocentesis for women in high risk groups. In a similar vein, euthanasia is now being explored as a viable option in cases of severe or prolonged suffering.

Several cultural values enter into these concerns. Our society believes that suffering is bad, that human life is good, that productive human beings are better than nonproductive ones, that it is good to support those in society who cannot support themselves and that all of us should earn our keep. Believing all of these things at once throws us into a moral dilemma, for some of them are incompatible with the others. We are a schizophrenic culture, for the same society which aborts a "fetus" or the "products of conception" also sells shirts for pregnant women with "BABY" written in big bold letters over the abdomen. Cultural values alone are inadequate to define humanity.

While cultural values are inadequate to determine our ethical decision making, they are part of us and must be examined. That examination process can be painful, especially for the Christian whose faith has become intertwined with the culture within which that faith was nurtured. For example, a group of Christian nurses were discussing the possibility of a union organizing in their hospital. Most were strongly against the union, feeling that it violated their Christian beliefs. Then one nurse spoke up, "My father was a union leader. I always thought the union members were the good guys and the nonunion workers were the unethical ones! For me, to be a Christian has been almost synonymous with being a union member."

Another problem in clarifying the personal context of ethical dilemmas is poor interpersonal communications. Sometimes we confuse a communications problem with an ethical dilemma. For instance, a nurse who refused to give a medication she felt was unsafe was fired. She felt that her right to question the doctor's order had been denied, so she contacted the district nurses association and asked them to defend her against the hospital. However, the reason she was fired was not that she had questioned the order, but because she had refused to give the medication without notifying the physician. The medication was a starting dose of digoxin, a higher dose than the nurse, who was relatively inexperienced, was accustomed to giving. She had written "NG" to signify "not given" beside the dose in the medicine Kardex but failed to explain to the next shift that she had not given the digoxin. The subsequent medicine nurses assumed that "NG" were the initials of the former medicine nurse and proceeded to give maintenance doses as ordered. In the meantime the patient's congestive heart failure was becoming more severe. The physician, assuming the patient had received all the medication as ordered, was preparing to take more drastic measures. The problem here was communication not ethics.

Gaining Objectivity

Every ethical dilemma is clouded by the influence of emotions, biases, values and communication problems. In order to clarify the real issues at stake, we need to become aware of our own responses and to determine the source of those attitudes and actions.

Do you find it difficult to care for certain types of patients? Try to identify what bothers you about them. Is there something you could do to overcome your feelings? For instance, if you dread caring for dying patients, would a workshop on death and dying be helpful? Or perhaps a Bible study with other nurses on the subject of death would enable you to work through some of your feelings. My own attitude toward child abusers has changed considerably through contact with an organization called "C.A.P.E." (Child Abuse Prevention Effort).

Personal biases can sometimes be overcome by receiving more accurate and adequate information, and most often that information comes from listening to the person whose behavior annoys you. For instance, the hepatitis patient I mentioned before was fearful and lonely. He had only recently begun to experiment with drugs because he felt that his parents and teachers would not listen to him and did not care about him. By ignoring his call light the nurse was only reinforcing his problem.

Cultural biases can be more difficult to correct because they are generally reinforced by the people around us. Dialog with people who disagree with you can help. If different sides of the issue are represented by Christians, a Bible study together on the subject could generate new understandings, even if the understanding is that it is all right to disagree.

One of the most painful learning experiences in my background came in the early seventies. I had been active in the civil rights movement in the sixties and saw myself as an unprejudiced crusader. Several years later at an InterVarsity summer camp some black Christians confronted me and the other whites present with, "You're prejudiced, all whites are!" After several days of hurt feelings and mounting anger the staff decided to have a panel of black students and staff address the camp with their feelings, followed by a panel of whites giving their response. Afterward, anger began to give way to understanding. The whites could begin to admit that we really did have a prejudice deeply ingrained in us by our culture. We could begin to say to our black brothers and sisters, "I'm sorry, please help me." They, in turn, could begin to understand our hurt and feelings of helplessness as we found our offers of fellowship and assistance rejected by them. We also learned that the first step in overcoming racial prejudice is to recognize it rather than deny it.

Finally, it is essential to follow proper channels of communication in clarifying the personal context of an ethical dilemma. Numerous ethical dilemmas have been created by nurses who rushed to the wrong people with inaccurate information because they felt threatened by what appeared to be a moral question. To move ahead crushing pride and overstepping the authority of persons along the way seldom solves an ethical dilemma. Poor communication fans tempers and stirs the fire, creating or exacerbating ethical dilemmas. A nurse who feels a moral obligation to self-righteously preach a particular ethical stance without adequate information seldom wins the case. Change comes about when nurses gently and firmly present an objective case with hard facts and clear alternatives.

For example, in a large state university hospital the nursing staff were deeply concerned because they felt patients were not receiving quality nursing care due to inadequate staffing. Most of the more experienced registered nurses had resigned to take positions in other hospitals where they felt they would have a better opportunity to give quality care. They had not been replaced. Tempers flared and there were rumors of a strike. Several Christian nurses on one unit suggested that a study be conducted to document their complaints, then presented to the nursing administration. The director of nursing was impressed by the thoroughness of their study and helped the nurses present their case to the hospital administration and later to the state authorities. The result, although not totally satisfactory, was a significant salary increase for all nursing personnel and institution of a unit manager system freeing nurses to spend more time with patients.

5
Defining the Problem

Step II. Define the Problem
A. Who is involved?
B. What issues are at stake?
C. What further information is needed?
1. biological
2. psychological
3. sociological
4. economic
5. legal
6. historical
7. philosophical
8. nursing standards

Suppose you're a registered nurse working on a general medical unit. Willie Barnes is one of your patients. He is fifty-seven years old, black and on welfare. An alcoholic with cirrhosis and chronic brain syndrome, he has no known family. He moves from boarding house to boarding house. He cannot read or write. He is frequently admitted to the hospital, usually brought in by the police when they find him unconscious in a public building or doorway. Willie seems to enjoy his stays; he relishes the food and attention. He is always very cooperative, but does not usually seem to fully comprehend verbal instructions.

One day as you are going through Willie's chart you discover a "living will" donating his corneas to the hospital when he dies. The document is signed with Willie's **X** and witnessed by an aide and the cleaning woman. You saw the ophthamology resident on the floor this morning. She is the wife of the medical resident who is assigned to Willie. You begin to suspect that Willie has signed something he does not understand.

Later you talk with the aide who witnessed the signing. She tells you that the resident came to talk to Willie while both she and the cleaning woman were in the room. The doctor told them about a young mother she had seen in the clinic who was going blind and could no longer care for her children. She said that Willie could give this young woman the gift of sight if he would sign the paper giving her his eyes after he died. The aide said that Willie was so happy he could help that he signed the paper with tears in his eyes.

Willie does not seem to recall signing the document, but he does say that a "pretty lady, a nice lady" came to talk to him. He seems to be quite pleased with the attention his visitor gave him and continues to talk about her. He says nothing of the living will or his eyes, even when questioned about the subjects.

Do you have a problem here? Willie is happy, and nobody, including Willie, is going to care if his corneas are removed after death. A young mother with keratoconus will be able to see again if she receives a corneal transplant. The ophthamology resident will gain valuable experience by having the opportunity to perform the surgery. Were Willie's rights really violated?

First, let's clarify the personal context. Emotionally, who tugs most at your sympathy? A semicoherent alcoholic who lives off public assistance with no family ties, or a vivacious young mother who is losing her vision? Are your emotions at all affected by the fact that Willie's physical condition was "self-imposed" through his drinking while the mother was a victim of a disease over which she had no control? Culturally, would you feel more protective of Willie if he were a white, retired businessman whose family had been killed in a car accident and whose brain damage was caused by a head injury? To clear up communications, where should you go to get the full story of what happened?

Now you are ready to begin defining the problem. The first step is to determine who is involved. Obviously Willie is, and so is the ophthamology resident. The aide and the cleaning woman who witnessed Willie's **X** are involved, but may not be aware of the ethical implications of their action. The woman with keratoconus has a definite stake in the situation, but probably does not know the source of the corneas she is scheduled to receive. You are involved now since you discovered the problem. Willie has no family, so it might appear that the effect of his "agreement" will be limited to the persons directly involved. But is that really the case? Each nurse who cares for Willie from now on will be involved. The quality of care he receives could be affected by the knowledge that he is scheduled to be a donor for a woman who needs his corneas as soon as possible. If this situation is allowed to pass unquestioned, future patients could be affected with more serious consequences. What superficially appeared to be a harmless agreement involving only three people is actually a dilemma with far-reaching effects.

The next step is to determine exactly what issues are at stake. We have already mentioned the care Willie might receive. To some people involved Willie is worth more dead than alive. If the sympathy of those caring for him is drawn toward the young mother, he might become the victim of negligence. More basic is the violation of his right to refuse to participate in the ophthamologist's plan. Although he "consented" by placing his **X** on the living will, he apparently did not understand what he was doing. He was not competent to make such a decision. Not only is Willie's own need for protection being violated, but the rights of other potential donors are at stake. If Willie can be coerced to sign a paper donating his corneas after death with no repercussions, then in the future another patient with limited understanding could be approached to request that he donate a vital organ while he is still alive. A far-reaching possibility is that mental institutions could become vast reservoirs for kidney donors.

Each issue at stake should be examined for its biological, psychological and sociological implications. In our society one prominent consideration is economic. A person supported by public funds may not receive equal treatment with the person who is affluent. Some people might rationalize the resident's action by saying that it costs the taxpayers thousands of dollars to keep Willie and the woman with keratoconus alive and fed, but if the young mother received Willie's corneas, she could once again support herself after her vision was restored. Knowing the cost of each alternative you might suggest in an ethical dilemma is important, even if you personally would not consider that a determining factor.

The legal aspects of a dilemma must be considered too. In this case, just what are Willie's legal rights? Are they being protected? History can often give a helpful perspective to a dilemma as well. In Willie's case you might explore how mentally incompetent persons have been treated in the past, how their treatment has changed over the years and the reasons for those changes. The philosophical rationale at work should be examined. Why did the resident feel it was appropriate to ask Willie to sign the living will? What values shaped her philosophy? Finally, you will need to describe the issues from a nursing perspective. What are your responsibilities as a nurse? Where can you intervene to change the situation? If nursing is caring and medicine is curing, how does Willie's situation become a specifically nursing concern?

6
Proposing and Evaluating Alternatives

Step III. Propose Alternatives
Step IV. Evaluate Alternatives
A.   Consider the effects and feasibility of each alternative
B.   Search the Scriptures
    1. determine patterns and principles from the whole of Scripture
    2. look up key words in a concordance and Bible dictionary
    3. look up problem passages in good commentaries
    4. examine the context of each passage to determine relevance
C.   Consult other Christians
    1. examine church history for precedents
    2. consult denominational statements
    3. read relevant materials by experts (theologians, ethicists)
    4. share your dilemma with a Bible study/prayer group
    5. ask advice of a more mature Christian nurse
    6. read books and articles by Christians who have faced similar dilemmas
D.   Decide which alternative is most in keeping with the character of God and the gospel of Jesus Christ

Once you have fully explored and defined the issues at stake you can begin to think about alternatives. Before getting caught up in evaluating the merit of each option, try to think of as many alternatives as you can. Just what could you do with Willie's situation? Write down whatever comes to mind, both the ridiculous as well as the practical ideas. For example, you could: not do anything, confront the ophthalmology resident with the problem, tell her husband you think the plan is unethical, tell the nursing supervisor about the problem, reprimand the aide and the cleaning woman who witnessed the signing of the living will, try to get Willie to rescind his permission, "leak" the story to an investigative reporter you know is concerned about civil rights, talk with other staff and try to get a solid group resistence to allowing the living will to be accepted as legal, get a lawyer involved, alert the hospital ethics committee, report the problem to the hospital administrator, ask the district nurses association for support or change jobs.

It helps to get others to brainstorm with you. Sometimes when you have exhausted all the possibilities in your own mind, a few ideas from other nurses can stimulate a whole series of new thoughts. Remember: this is not the time for evaluation of the ideas, but a time for opening up every course of action possible.

Brainstorming about alternatives to an ethical dilemma can be frustrating. Frequently we are left with the feeling that there are no choices, or that all the choices are bad. Now it is time to stop and ask again for the Lord's guidance. Take time to pray through the situation. Pray for Willie, asking God to help you know him as a person, to understand his needs, to care for him properly and lovingly, and to be able to represent him fairly. Pray for the resident, asking that the Lord will help you to hear her side of the problem with an open mind and to communicate with her rationally and calmly. Pray for each person involved in the situation, specifically and personally. Then pray about the issues and ask God's guidance for you as you think through alternatives. Ask that those involved would be able to come to the same conclusion, and that God would be glorified in the situation.

Now start evaluating alternatives. Consider the effects and feasibility of each alternative. One of the easiest solutions would be to just ignore the situation. That would avoid the pain of confrontation, and Willie wouldn't know the difference. Or would he? Would his care deteriorate? Would there be other patients later who would suffer because of the precedent set in this case?

A first step in taking action could be to talk to the resident about the situation giving reasons for your concern. She might be receptive to what you say and change her mind. Or she could become angry and proceed as planned, in which case you could take your concern to the nursing administration and keep appealing to higher administrative levels until you are satisfied with the response. You might endanger your job security if you make the wrong people angry, so you will need to have your facts in writing, well-researched and documented.

What if you go through all the proper channels with no response? Then it is time to re-evaluate. What reasons have the authorities given for their positions? Are they valid? Who are they protecting by refusing to take your concerns seriously? If you still feel that your position is correct, keep thinking of other options. Could you take it to the press? What would happen if the situation were exposed to the public? What if the story became distorted? Would the story destroy public confidence in the hospital? Is this situation worth that risk? Are there other options? Could you gain support through your district nurses association? Would contacting a lawyer be helpful? How much would it cost? Who would pay? If similar dilemmas frequently occur at this hospital, should you consider changing jobs? How would that help Willie?

Whatever you do in proposing alternatives, don't stop at two or three. If you get stumped, stop and pray some more. Talk with other nurses.

Keep thinking. There is always more than one solution. Your goal should be to find the best solution—not the only one. Now you are ready to search the Scriptures for further help in evaluating your alternatives.

God's Will and the Bible

Although most nurses routinely use analytical thinking in the nursing process, for some reason decisions about faith and morals are usually based on pat formulas. We want the Bible to provide those formulas and may become defensive if someone implies that it does not. Consider the following questions, then look up the references given:

Would you refuse to allow a person to worship with you if his grandmother was illegitimate? (Deut. 23:2)

Would you refuse to work (as a nurse) on Sunday? (Ex. 20:8; Lk. 14:1-6)

Would you deny your faith if your parents told you to? (Ex. 20:12; Mt. 10:34-37)

If you are a woman, would you refuse to teach men? (1 Tim. 2:12; Acts 18:26)

Do you always cover your head to pray? (1 Cor. 11:5)

Do you ever wear gold necklaces? (1 Pet. 3:3)

Your answers probably demonstrate that you are selective in your use of Scripture. There are good reasons for that selectivity, but most Christians are not aware of them. Most of us have merely accepted our parents', our denomination's, or our pastor's interpretation of Scripture and have never done much thinking about how they arrived at their conclusions. Then, in the process of using the Bible to find ethical guidelines, all sorts of problems arise. We pull out isolated passages and build ethical conclusions on them, or become discouraged when conflicting directions are given, or feel that the Bible gives no direction at all if the specific modern dilemma we are facing is not discussed.

Most people want ethical guidelines in the form of rules or laws. It is easier that way, since being able to follow a law relieves the individual from the agony of personal decision. But the Bible presents us with a tension between law and gospel. The law is God's rulebook which tells us how far we have strayed from his desires for us. The gospel is the good news of forgiveness and redemption in Christ which frees us to do his will. We learn God's will by prayerfully studying the Bible and by daily living in relationship to God. The law does not embody the fullness of God's will. Klaus Bockmuehl suggests, "The Ten Commandments are like the safety rails on a motorway, protecting the driver from the abyss or uncertain ground to his right or left, and one is surely grateful for them. On the other hand no one would wish to drive his car, steering wheel locked, solely by the means of those safety rails."[1] If the law is the guard-rails, then the gospel is the road we want to follow.

The relationship between the law and the gospel and the effect of that relationship is the core of Christian ethics. The law sets the outer boundaries of the permissible; the gospel makes a relationship with God possible so we can do what pleases him. Therefore, if we look to the law alone for our ethical guidelines, we have missed the point. On the other hand, we are sinners and our love is not perfect, so we cannot disregard the law and "do the most loving thing" in each situation. Our human nature clouds our ability to accurately and fairly determine what the most loving action would be. We need an outside authority and clear guidelines to clarify the form our love must take.

The Christian's authority is God himself, so one of our ethical guidelines is to consider whether a certain alternative is in keeping with the character of God. An understanding of God's character cannot be gained from a few short prooftexts, but must be gleaned from years of consistent prayer, Bible study and day-to-day living in relationship to God. Since our relationship with God is dependent on his grace toward us in the gospel of Jesus Christ, not on our ability to keep the law, we can rest assured that our salvation is not dependent on our ethics; however, our ethics should certainly be affected by our salvation. It is all right for two sincere Christians to arrive at different conclusions to the same dilemma if the Bible is silent or ambiguous about the issue. God does not call us to be right all the time. He calls us to be faithful; and he forgives us when we are faithfully wrong.

When the Bible Is Unclear

At times the Bible seems to give clear enough guidelines on both sides of an issue to cause Christians to reach opposite conclusions. An example is the Christian's relationship to secular authority. Some claim that secular authority must be obeyed at all cost, up to, but not including, denying one's faith. They use Romans 13:1-7 and Mark 12:13-17 to back up their position. Others, using Acts 5:29, claim no allegiance to authorities whom they consider to be unjust or unethical.

Many major issues in nursing ethics are never mentioned in the Bible. The question of whether to artificially prolong life was not a problem in Bible times; it was not possible. Unions are not mentioned because they did not exist. Only one ambiguous text refers to abortions (Exodus 21: 22-25). One passage has been occasionally quoted out of context to demonstrate that the Bible is against euthanasia (2 Samuel 1:1-16). However, although specific case studies of ethical dilemmas identical to yours may not be found in Scripture, the Bible is quite clear about God's concern for justice, mercy and the sanctity of life. To make decisions in such cases we must look at the whole of Scripture to determine what actions would be most in keeping with the character of God.

The Bible is a big book. Where does a person begin to discover what would be pleasing to God? Let's say that your health agency has voted to unionize registered nurses. You are not sure how you feel about the plan. Several other Christian nurses have told you that they will resign when the union membership becomes mandatory. You wonder what you should do. First, you will need to clarify the personal context and define the problem accurately, propose alternatives and then begin to search for patterns and principles in Scripture which might indicate God's will for you.

Suppose you identified the issues at stake as : (1) your responsibility to patients, (2) your loyalty to your employer and (3) fairness in hospital employment practices. To find out what the Bible has to say on these subjects a good starting point would be a concordance. Try to think of all the key words related to the issues and possible biblical synonyms. For example:

responsibility—faithfulness, loyalty, duty, trust
patients—sick, infirm, oppressed, diseased, poor, sheep, neighbor
loyalty—submission, obedience, service, duty, honor
employer—shepherd, master, steward, elder, authority
fairness—justice, virtue, stewardship, due wages, family needs and responsibilities, oppression, deceive

Now begin looking up the words. Some of the passages which contain the words may not apply at all; others may seem conflicting or unclear. Make a list of all the ones which seem applicable, even if they do not all appear to agree. When your list is complete, turn to some good commentaries, which take the original languages into consideration, to clarify any passages which seem unclear. You may be dealing with two or more Greek or Hebrew words with different meanings which have been translated by the same English word. For example, the Greek words *agape* and *philia* are both translated "love." Commentaries will also help to put the passages into the context of the culture for which they were originally intended.

Another way of understanding passages which seem to conflict is to look at the Old Testament in the light of the New. For instance, the command in Leviticus 20:10 to stone anyone caught in the act of adultery is softened by Jesus' treatment of the woman at the well in John 4:7-26. A Bible dictionary will be helpful at this point. Look up the same key words to find a summary of most of the major uses of each with comments on its theological implications.

In the long run the union question could be reduced to applying the command to "love your neighbor as yourself." But that is not such a simple matter when your neighbor includes your employer, patients, colleagues and your own family, each with different demands upon your loyalty. Old Testament patterns of justice, and New Testament guidelines for relationships need to be applied in the context of your present situation. To a large extent your decision will be determined by how you perceive the importance of the issues at stake. The Bible will shape your understanding of justice and relationships, but the methods by which justice is attained and loving relationships are nurtured will depend on the way you view the dilemma.

Let's apply this process to our situation with Willie and the young mother with keratoconus. Here the basic issue is informed consent, a concept about which there is no specific biblical teaching. We have identified one of the related issues to be quality of care. The amount of time and concern spent on Willie might quickly deteriorate if he were worth more dead than alive to some people involved. Overshadowing the whole picture is the fact that Willie is poor and black. Now some key words begin to take shape for our consideration:

poor—oppressed, downtrodden, weak, feeble, afflicted, destitute, needy, hungry, naked

care (of sick)—healing, nurse, nurture, bind up, nourish, shepherd, infirm, diseased, neighbor

justice—righteousness, judge, equity, reward, punishment

A quick survey of passages containing the word *poor* in a concordance reveals that poor people hold a special place in God's heart. References are numerous and almost all of them speak in favor of the poor. One passage seems to condone not liking the poor when read by itself. Proverbs 14:20 says, "The poor is disliked even by his neighbor, but the rich has many friends." But read in context, this passage presents a strong case for the poor, for the following verse says, "He who despises his neighbor is a sinner, but happy is he who is kind to the poor." Exodus 23:3 seems to be an unusual verse when compared with other passages about the poor, "Nor shall you be partial to a poor man in his suit." When read in context it still seems a bit out of character with the rest of the passage. By looking up the passage in a commentary we find that there is a strong possibility that a similar Hebrew word meaning "a powerful man" could have been in the original text, or else it could have been intended to communicate that no one, rich or poor, should automatically be considered right because of his economic status.[2]

The article "Poverty" in *The New Bible Dictionary* (Grand Rapids: Eerdmans, 1962) summarizes the biblical teaching about the poor in the Old and New Testaments. The Old Testament, especially, focuses on the responsibility of the rich to care for the poor. The New Testament speaks more of the benefit of being materially poor, and the dangers of being rich. The article points out key passages and briefly explains the message of each. A Bible dictionary may provide direction and theological insights on a topic, but it is no substitute for studying the actual Bible passages yourself. You will probably gain a deeper feeling for God's concern for the poor by reading what the Bible says firsthand, than by reading what someone else says it says.

After you have exhausted your resources on the word "poor," you are ready to move on to the next word on your list. There is always the temptation to come to a conclusion quickly, but remember, our goal is to consider all aspects of the problem so that we will find God's will in the situation.

Reading in Context

Literary context is extremely important when using the Bible for ethical decision making. Everything from slavery to shunning electricity have been defended by sincere Christians who used Scripture out of context. The most basic safeguard in determining context is to read the passages before and after an isolated verse. What is the frame of reference? What reasons are given for that particular advice? Does it seem to be a universal principle or a solution to a unique problem? Who is giving the advice? I once sat through a lengthy group Bible study where the leader was using the advice of Job's comforters as a guideline for meeting patient's spiritual needs. She had not read far enough in the book of Job to discover that God condemned the help given by Job's friends.

Beyond the literary context, it is also important to look at the geographical and cultural context. What was the situation of the people being addressed in a particular passage? Were they Jews in exile who thought they had left God behind in Jerusalem? Were they gentile Christians surrounded by pagan influences? Were they Jewish Christians who felt uncomfortable without the law? For instance, when you read Colossians it is helpful to know something about the Gnostics in order to understand Paul's advice. 1 Corinthians may seem to give some conflicting rules about women unless you understand first-century attitudes and customs concerning women.

Ethical admonitions in the New Testament are not given as a new law, but as interpretations of the gospel's effects on everyday life. Therefore, in order to fully understand and apply the principles contained in them we need to look at the context in which they originally applied. Examining Scripture in context does not mean that we can gloss over moral guidelines or dismiss major admonitions as "time-conditioned." It does mean that we must take seriously all the factors involved so that we can responsibly apply the gospel to our own lives.

In the Bible we have God's word in written form, yet our knowledge of God's will remains imperfect and incomplete. We don't have all the answers. We are going to make mistakes. Yet God expects us to represent him in the world. We have to speak out for justice and mercy in society as we perceive it. That is what faith is all about. Faith is a dynamic relationship with the living God. It is learning obedience step by step through trial and error. Although the process may seem painful and tedious, we can be grateful that God loves us and nurtures us as individuals rather than providing us with a built-in computer program for righteous living.

What we have learned about the character of God through reading and studying the Bible over the years will provide both a foundation and a measuring rod for our in-depth Bible study concerning ethical issues. Our basic working knowledge of the Scriptures provides us with an overview of patterns and principles for Christian living. Over the years our intuitive sense of right and wrong should be molded through Sunday school, personal Bible study, group Bible studies, sermons and other exposures to God's people and his Word. As we reflect on what we know about the Bible as a whole, we will develop an ability to discern God's voice in particular situations. When we hear something which seems out of character for the Lord—even if it comes from Scripture—our knowledge of the whole of Scripture acts as a measuring rod which sends us back to double-check for context and interpretations.

How the Church Can Help

One conclusion we can draw from a study of the Bible as a whole is that God has invested the church and its leaders with wisdom and authority (Mt. 16:16-19; Gal. 2:1-2; Eph. 3:8-10; 1 Thess. 5:12-13; 1 Tim. 3:14-15; Tit. 1:1-3; 2:15). The church provides several resources in ethical decision making when the Bible appears to be silent or unclear on an issue.

Church history provides one source of illumination. For example, the Bible has no clear, specific teaching about abortion, even though it was a common practice in the Greco-Roman world of the first century.[3] The church condemned abortion from the beginning. The *Didache,* one of the earliest manuals of church instruction, states, "Thou shalt not procure abortion, nor commit infanticide."[4] The *Epistle of Barnabas,* a document from the late first, or early second century states, "Thou shalt love thy neighbor more than thy own life. Thou shalt not procure abortion, thou shalt not commit infanticide."[5] In the early third century Tertullian wrote, "For us, indeed, as homicide is forbidden, it is not lawful to destroy what is conceived in the womb while the blood is still being formed into a man. To prevent being born is to accelerate homicide, nor does it make a difference whether you snatch away a soul which is born or destroy one being born. He who is man-to-be is man, as all fruit is now in the seed."[6]

The position of the church remained unwaivering for over a thousand years. About the twelfth century some church leaders supported making a few exceptions to preserve the health of the mother. At that time many of the same questions asked today were introduced: When does the fetus become human? When does the soul enter the embryo? Is abortion murder? Does the unborn baby have a right to life if its birth would cause the mother's death? By the eighteenth century the Roman Catholic Church resumed its firm stand against abortion, while most Protestant churches continued to wrestle with the issue.

Church history does not hold equal authority with Scripture for the evangelical Christian. If it did we would end up in total confusion. We can, however, learn from what has been done in the past. The situation in the non-Christian Greco-Roman world was similar to our own in many ways. Abortions were popularly practiced for reasons of convenience. The firm stand of the Christian church against abortion presented a marked contrast to society's norms. The reasons given by the church for its stand were: (1) that we should love our neighbors, including unborn neighbors, (2) that we should respect what God has created and (3) that the fetus is human. Thus the weight of Christian opinion historically falls on the antiabortion side.

Another source of guidance from the church is the official statements of denominational bodies. Most denominations have committees of theologians who study social problems and attempt to apply the teachings of Scripture to them. Social statements and position papers can usually be obtained from your pastor or from your denominational headquarters.

The writings of theologians and ethicists, both past and present, can further inform us for making ethical decisions. You may find it especially helpful to read several authors with differing viewpoints. Even if you do not agree with their theology or their conclusions, each may have some good arguments. Paul Ramsey, though theologically liberal, is a relatively conservative ethicist concentrating in bioethics. Near the other end of the spectrum is Joseph Fletcher, famous for his *Situation Ethics,* who has also done extensive work in the same field. Helmut Thielicke is an outstanding German Lutheran ethicist with evangelical commitments. Carl Henry, a leading American evangelical, has written extensively on ethics. The church at large has become deeply concerned about the problems involved in bioethical decision making. We can look forward to a wealth of material being published in the future.

The church is also composed of lay persons. The experiences of other Christians who are facing the same or similar dilemmas can provide further resources. If several Christians are involved in a dilemma, you might want to meet together for prayer and Bible study about the problem. For instance, if we go back to the question about joining a union, each individual Christian could decide on a different action for different reasons. But if those persons got together and shared their feelings and rationales, perhaps they could explore new alternatives and see a fuller view of what the Bible has to say about the issues at stake. If you are feeling alone in your concern about a particular dilemma, you might want to discuss the problem with an older, more experienced Christian nurse who has faced similar situations in the past. Books by Christian nurses, physicians, lawyers, paramedical personnel and patients cover a wide range of ethical dilemmas. Their personal insights can also help to direct our thinking.

Christian ethics can never be merely a private decision process. First of all, because other people will be affected by our decisions, then also because we need the wisdom and insights of other Christians to evaluate and balance our own conclusions.

for further reading:
Bible Study Aids:
Concordance to the Holy Bible. American Bible Society, 1960.
Food for Life. Peter Lee, Greg Scharf, Robert Willcox. IVP, 1977, pp. 146-51.
How to Study the Bible. Edited by John B. Job. IVP, 1972, pp. 83-90.
The Jerome Biblical Commentary. Edited by Raymond E. Brown, Joseph Fitzmyer and Roland Murphy. Prentice-Hall, 1968.
The New Bible Commentary: Revised. Edited by D. Guthrie, J. A. Motyer,

A. M. Stibbs and D. J. Wiseman. IVP, 1970.
The New Bible Dictionary. Edited by J. D. Douglas. IVP, 1962.
The RSV Handy Concordance. Zondervan, 1962.

Books on Guidance:
Barclay, Oliver R. *Guidance.* IVP, 1978.
Bayly, Joseph, and others. *His Essays on Guidance.* IVP, 1968.
Little, Paul. *Affirming the Will of God.* IVP, 1971.
Mumford, Bob. *Take Another Look at Guidance.* Logos, 1971.
Redpath, Alan. *Getting to Know the Will of God.* IVP, 1954.
Smith, M. Blaine. *Knowing God's Will.* IVP, 1979.

7
Taking Action

Step V. Develop a Plan of Action

A. Prepare for confrontation
1. collect data
2. document data in writing
3. be prepared to support alternatives with facts and rationale
4. contact all persons involved in decision making
5. determine who has power to effect change and enlist them in the decision-making process
6. find prayer support
7. double-check your motives and attitudes

B. Move into action
1. go directly and privately to persons involved
2. own your opinions
3. confront without placing blame or attacking the person's character
4. be objective and specific
5. listen to the other side of the story
6. be willing to change your opinions
7. go through proper channels

Ethical decision making is only useful if it leads to action. Careful planning is necessary to assure that the action is responsible and effective. Data should be collected and documented in writing. You should be prepared to support proposed alternatives with facts and rationale. All persons who will be involved in carrying out the ethical behavior need to be contacted and involved in the decisions made. You will need to determine who has the power to effect change and then to enlist those persons in the decision-making process. Finally, you will need faithful prayer support.

For an example, let's say that you are being oriented to a new unit in a medical center. The unit is equipped with a Brewer system, so you can obtain drugs from a machine by inserting the patient's charge card along with the plate for a specific prescription drug. You are giving medicines on the evening shift for the first time when the charge nurse tells you that since most of the patients receive Dalmane for sleep you can save time by pulling several boxes of Dalmane using the first few patients' charge cards. You can then keep the boxes on top of the medicine cart so they will be handy to give to all the patients receiving Dalmane. You mention that it doesn't seem fair for a few patients to be paying for the medication given to others. She replies, "Well, we don't always use the same patients' charge cards. We try to rotate it. Anyway, the insurance companies pay the bills; the patients don't."

You go through the steps of the decision-making process in your mind and come to the conclusion that the practice of giving borrowed Dalmane is wrong. Now you can begin to formulate a plan. First you need to collect data and document it in writing. Find out the cost of the Dalmane. A little capsule doesn't look expensive; perhaps the nurses giving it feel that the cost is negligible. They might be impressed with the seriousness of their action if they knew the actual cost. Look on the patients' charts to see how many are actually covered by insurance. Often we assume that all our patients are covered when they are not. Consider what the added burden might be on people who have no insurance and find themselves charged with medications they did not receive. Next, look at some insurance company figures to see if such waste and overcharging result in significant rate increases. Write down all your information.

After you have collected the facts, examine the alternatives you have proposed in the light of the same type of data. For instance, if you were to determine a slow period in the evening when you could routinely check each patient's drawer to see if a fresh supply of Dalmane and other medications is needed and restock, would that save as much or more time? Time yourself a couple of times to see. Or if the day shift, who is supposed to do the restocking, were reminded to stock Dalmane for each patient for whom it is ordered, could the problem be eliminated? Or if hospital policy is not to stock p.r.n. drugs in advance, could an exception be made for Dalmane and other drugs patients use on a regular basis? In each case, the reason the problem developed in the first place must be considered and addressed. Time and convenience seem to be the root causes.

The broader problem would not be solved at all if you merely decided that you would not continue the practice. Too many other nurses are involved. Each nurse who gives medicines on the evening shift may be following the charge nurse's instructions to borrow Dalmane. You will need to convince each of them that the practice is unethical.

In this case, who has the power to change the situation? You are new on the unit. You are one of several staff nurses. You can suggest and inform, but you have no actual power. Individual nurses have the power to change their own behavior, but they need leadership. Convincing the charge nurse of the need for change appears to be the most direct and effective means of solving the problem. If she is unresponsive, the head nurse may need to take responsibility for correcting the situation.

As you formulate your plan several sources of possible tension and antagonism will become evident. None of us want to be told that we are being unethical. None of us like criticism. Few people will want to change a way of doing something which feels comfortable and convenient. A strong prayer base is essential for you as you move from the planning stage to acting on your plan. Ask several people to pray for you—that you would have sensitivity and tact when you confront the individuals involved in the unethical practices. Also ask them to pray for the persons involved—that they would be willing to hear what you have to say and consider alternative ways of dispensing the Dalmane.

Once your plan is complete and you have enlisted prayer support, stop and review your plans prayerfully, double-checking your motives and your attitudes. Consider whether you have earned the right to be heard. In this case you are a newcomer to the unit. Have you established enough rapport with your coworkers for them to trust you and respect your opinions? Can you identify with their need to save time in dispensing medicines? Have you been fair in evaluating their priorities? For instance, is the time they save in giving out the bedtime sedations being used for more important functions? Is it allowing them to be more accurate and less rushed in passing out medications? What are your motives? Are you actually concerned about increased cost to the patients, or are you trying to impress your supervisor with your honesty? Are you earnestly trying to be fair, or are you rigidly adhering to the rules because they are rules? Are you hoping to improve the quality of care given by all nurses on your unit, or are you wanting others to see you as the "supernurse" who always does things right because she's a Christian.

Moving into Action

If you decide that your motives are good and your attitude is humble and concerned, then you are ready to move into action. First, *go directly and privately to the person or persons involved.* Jesus said, "If your brother sins against you, go and tell him his fault, between you and him alone. If he listens to you, you have gained your brother. But if he does not listen, take one or two others along with you, that every word may be confirmed by the evidence of two or three witnesses" (Mt. 18:15-16). Going alone conveys trust and respect. It gives people the opportunity to tell their side of the story, to explain their rationale. It allows them to change their behavior without losing face. It gives them a fair chance to dispute your charges. If you bring along reinforcements from the beginning, you put yourself at an unfair advantage.

Another way of ganging up on the person you are confronting is to say, "A lot of people think this is unethical," or, "Several of us have decided that this practice should be discontinued." Avoid this when you confront a person by *owning your opinions.* Say, *"I'm* concerned that patients are being charged for drugs they don't use," or, *"I* think it would be better if we pulled a box of Dalmane for each patient who uses it and dispense it accordingly so that patients will only be charged for what they use."

By owning your opinions you can also *confront without placing blame or attacking the character* of the person involved. Be *objective and specific,* giving simple, clear facts without exaggerating their importance or moralizing. Present your information about the cost of the Dalmane, the number of patients without insurance, the increases in insurance rates resulting for overcharging and waste. Assume that the person has the best of motives until proven otherwise. In other words, don't say something like, "Boy, that's really a sloppy way to give medications!" This is also not the time for quoting Scripture in an accusing manner, like, "He who walks in integrity walks securely, but he who perverts his ways will be found out" (Prov. 10:9). If you truly hope to "gain your brother," you have to remain on his side, even while you are questioning what he is doing.

After you have presented your case, *listen to the other person's side of the story.* That person may have information you don't have. Perhaps a rationale was developed in response to a unique problem on the unit before you came. Maybe Dalmane is a stock drug for which patients are not charged. *Be willing to change your opinions* if the other person presents evidence which is contrary to your information.

But suppose you are still not satisfied after going through all of the above steps. In the process of confronting individuals you discover that the practice is much more widespread than you had imagined. Not only Dalmane but also antibiotics and other drugs which are commonly ordered are being pooled and given from a common box. Drugs left after a patient is discharged, which are supposed to be counted and credited to his account, are also pooled into common boxes. Not only are patients being charged for drugs they did not use, but errors are being made. In one box of ampicillin lying on the medicine cart you found a mixture of 250 mg. and 500 mg. capsules. The box is labeled "250 mg." The only thing left to do is to "take one or two others with you."

In that case it is extremely important that you *go through proper channels*. Think through the authority structure of your agency and your list of people who have power to change things. You might get plenty of action if you began telling attending physicians that their patients are being overcharged because of the lazy practices of medicine nurses, but you would also create an explosive situation. Doctors and nurses would be at odds with one another. Instead, choose the person next in authority over those you have confronted. In this case that would most likely be the head nurse. Again, present specific, objective facts without attacking the character of the persons involved. Only after going through the entire chain of command without achieving satisfaction should you turn to an outside source of pressure such as the media or a consumer advocate. But if all else fails, you could write a letter to the editor of your local paper suggesting that patients check their hospital bills carefully and question any items listed which they did not receive.

In the process of gathering data and acting on your ethical decisions, remember that you are a nurse and not an investigative reporter. While it is important to maintain high ethical standards, it is also important to maintain congenial working relationships in order to give safe and compassionate nursing care. We must take action carefully and gently, considering the needs and feelings of the persons involved in what we perceive as unethical behavior. We need to promote an atmosphere of trust and openness where constructive criticism can be offered without crushing tender feelings. We also need to communicate an openness to receive criticism as well as to criticize. High ethical standards can be consistently maintained only in a milieu of mutuality and support.

for further reading:
Alexander, John W. *Practical Criticism,* IVP, 1976.
Augsburger, David. *Caring Enough to Confront.* Regal, 1973.

8
A Case Study in Applying the Decision-Making Process

Do not deceive yourselves by just listening
to his word; instead, put it into
practice.... Whoever looks closely
into the perfect law that sets people
free, who keeps on paying attention to it
and does not simply listen and then
forget it, but puts it into practice—that
person will be blessed by God in
what he does.
James 1:22, 25 (Good News Bible)

Is the decision-making process proposed here really practical for ethical dilemmas? Will it work in the tangled situations you find yourself struggling with? So far we have looked at examples of each aspect of the decision-making process. Now it is time to put it all together. The following case study will give us the opportunity to look at the whole process in action.

Case Study

Sally Miller was charge nurse on a surgical unit where Mrs. Barbara Schwartz was transferred after two weeks on a medical unit. Mrs. Schwartz, a fifty-six-year-old Jewish homemaker who looked closer to forty than sixty, had a year ago undergone a hysterectomy for carcinoma of the uterus. She assumed that she had been cured at that time. Experiencing some mild gastrointestinal upset she had re-entered the hospital for tests. The tests proved suspicious so surgery was indicated. When the attending physician explained the need for surgery to Mr. and Mrs. Schwartz, they became angry and hostile toward the doctor and nursing personnel. At this point Mrs. Schwartz was transferred to Sally's unit. The charge nurse from the medical unit called to report on the transfer, concluding her remarks with, "Good luck, we're glad to get rid of her!"

Both Mr. and Mrs. Schwartz exhibited a great deal of anxiety nonverbally but maintained an everything-is-fine attitude around each other. Mr. Schwartz often paced the corridor while Mrs. Schwartz slept, wringing his hands and muttering critical comments to nursing personnel as he passed them in the hall. He hired private duty nurses around the clock, and Mrs. Schwartz fired them in rapid succession.

Mrs. Schwartz was scheduled for surgery, but it had to be postponed twice. Each morning of the day surgery was scheduled Mrs. Schwartz went into respiratory distress so surgery had to be delayed until a pulmonary embolus could be ruled out. After each episode she refused to sign another operative permit. The surgeon finally became impatient and scheduled Mrs. Schwartz for the operating room about a week later, hoping she would relent and sign the permit. She reluctantly agreed to sign if she could have a psychiatric consultation before surgery.

On the evening before surgery Sally sat with Mrs. Schwartz while her private duty nurse was at dinner. She helped Mrs. Schwartz verbalize her fears, then offered to pray for her. A deep, trusting relationship was initiated at that time. As it was, Sally did not respect most of the private duty nurses in the registry, but now she began to resent them. She felt that they were not providing Mrs. Schwartz with quality nursing care.

Surgery revealed metastatic carcinoma of the large and small bowel and the liver. After the surgeon informed Mr. and Mrs. Schwartz about the diagnosis, their hostile behavior intensified. They hired and fired private duty nurses more rapidly, continually called the nursing office to report floor personnel for incompetence and threatened to sue the physicians.

Their relationship to Sally, though, continued to be good. They trusted her and would agree to almost anything she suggested. Each of them poured out their fears, guilt and frustrations to Sally. Mrs. Schwartz said she had not felt like a woman after her hysterectomy. Her husband had treated her coolly; he seemed afraid to get close to her. She said that she could find no meaning and purpose to life if she could not be completely well. She would rather die than be an invalid. Mr. Schwartz, a prominent lawyer, confessed to Sally that he was seeing another woman. The affair began after his wife's hysterectomy. His girl friend came with him each day to the hospital and waited in the cafeteria. Mr. Schwartz said that it was important to him to have a "beautiful and vivacious woman" at his side at social functions. Mrs. Schwartz had not been able to fulfill that role since her surgery. Yet now he felt that he could not bear to see her suffer. He continually asked Sally to give his wife "something that will take her out of her misery permanently." (The private duty nurse was not qualified to give medications.) Each time he asked, Sally refused.

A week after surgery Mr. Schwartz employed a new private duty nurse who was qualified to give medications. Mrs. Schwartz seemed to like her. This nurse was very protective of Mrs. Schwartz and became hostile to Sally whenever she entered Mrs. Schwartz's room or requested to see the chart. The chart was supposed to be kept at the nurses' station, but this private duty nurse insisted on keeping it in the patient's room. At first she refused to report to Sally at the end of the day, but would only report to the oncoming private duty nurse. At Sally's insistence and appeal to hospital policy (which private duty nurses were required to abide by), she finally began reporting to her as well. Her reports were vague and incomplete. She kept intake and output records on scraps of paper and refused to put them on the chart until after Sally had read it. When Sally asked for the figures the nurse replied, "I don't have them yet." Sally complained to the supervisor about the private duty nurse's behavior. The supervisor responded that she was the last nurse in the registry left to call and that Sally would have to put up with her. "I'm tired of catering to these Jewish prima donnas. I've had it!" she told Sally. Sally insisted that she felt that the nurse was unsafe. The supervisor told her to document her complaint.

Over the next week the problem grew worse. Mrs. Schwartz appeared dehydrated and lethargic. She was receiving p.r.n. morphine every two hours, although she stated that she had no pain and did not want the injections. Her respirations were obviously very slow, yet were recorded as normal on the chart. Her intake and output were always recorded as normal, but the Foley drainage bag was almost empty each time Sally checked on Mrs. Schwartz. Her skin and mouth appeared dry. The private duty nurse became even more vague and evasive in response to Sally's questions. Finally Sally entered the patient's room as the nurse was giving her a drink of water. The suction machine attached to Mrs. Schwartz's Levine tube was set on high and quickly drained the liquid into the bottle. Sally asked the nurse to come to the nurses' station. There she reminded the private duty nurse that the Levine tube was supposed to be clamped for two hours after eating or drinking, and asked her how often she had left it open while feeding Mrs. Schwartz. "The doctor gave me verbal orders to leave it unclamped at all times," she responded.

"Her husband wants her dead, and she doesn't have anything to live for anyway."

A quick phone call confirmed the physician's verbal order to leave the Levine tube unclamped. He said, "I'm respecting the family's wishes to let the lady die in peace."

Sally felt angry and bewildered. She tried to explain to the physician that Mrs. Schwartz was not ready to die—she still had emotional and spiritual tasks to complete—and that Mr. Schwartz seemed to have other motives besides compassion for wanting her dead. The surgeon laughed at her. ■

Deciding What to Do

Put yourself in Sally's place. What would you be feeling at this point? How would you begin to discern God's will for this situation? What decisions need to be made?

First, let's review the decision-making process:

Step I. Clarify the Personal Context
A. Identify emotional responses
B. Explore personal biases
C. Examine cultural values
D. Open interpersonal communication

Step II. Define the Probelm
A. Who is involved?
B. What issues are at stake?
C. What further information is needed?
    1. biological
    2. psychological
    3. sociological
    4. economic
    5. legal
    6. historical
    7. philosophical
    8. nursing standards

Step III. Propose Alternatives
Step IV. Evaluate Alternatives
A. Consider the effects and feasibility of each alternative

B. Search the Scriptures
    1. determine patterns and principles from the whole of Scripture
    2. look up key words in a concordance and Bible dictionary
    3. look up problem passages in good commentaries
    4. examine the context of each passage to determine relevance
C. Consult other Christians
    1. examine church history for precedents
    2. consult denominational statements
    3. read relevant materials by the experts (theologians and ethicists)
    4. share your dilemma with a Bible study/prayer group
    5. ask advice of a more mature Christian nurse
    6. read books and articles by Christians who have faced similar dilemmas
D. Decide which alternative is most in keeping with the character of God and the gospel of Jesus Christ

Step V. Develop a Plan of Action

Now let's apply it to the Schwartz case.

Step I: Clarifying the Personal Context

Emotional Responses. Almost every ethical dilemma will be contaminated with emotional reactions, and this one is no exception. Mr. and Mrs. Schwartz made life so miserable for hospital personnel that few, if any, could relate to them in an objective manner. How would you feel toward someone who had reported you for incompetence, or caused you a great deal of extra work, or fired you?

The private duty nurse who was suspected of unethical conduct may have been afraid of being fired too. To protect her job she may have felt she needed to be particularly attentive and protective, and to do anything she was asked by Mr. or Mrs. Schwartz or the physician in charge. She may have been swept up into the emotional climate of the Schwartzes and seen herself as their only true ally in a hostile environment.

Sally may also have felt that she was their only ally. She had a personal stake in the dilemma since she had been able to establish rapport with Mrs. Schwartz, but had been cut off from the relationship by the presence of the private duty nurse. A personal power struggle contaminated her objectivity.

Mrs. Schwartz was afraid of death and the disease process. She was so desperately afraid of being alone that she set up a defense system which kept people away. She could not even be honest with her husband. She felt alienated and lonely.

Mr. Schwartz was a caldron of emotions. He was filled with guilt over his illicit affair, fear of his wife's death, anger over her illness preventing him from living his carefree social life, grief over her suffering and impatience to get it all over with so life could go back to normal.

The nursing supervisor had little personal contact with Mrs. Schwartz. She knew her as the "problem on 6 East" who had gone through every private duty nurse in the registry, whose husband called daily to complain about floor personnel and every department in the hospital which provided services for his wife. She knew that Mr. Schwartz was influential in the community, and she was concerned about the bad publicity the hospital might receive from him. Mrs. Schwartz was not a person in need to her; she was an emotional threat.

The attending physician was also frustrated by Mrs. Schwartz. He had to postpone surgery twice. He had not been able to cure his patient. He experienced her hostility. He may have felt intimidated by her lawyer husband. Mr. Schwartz's insistence that Mrs. Schwartz be taken out of her misery may have been feeding into the physician's sense of frustration and helplessness.

Personal Biases. Sally did not respect most of the private duty nurses in the registry. Her distrust of private duty nurses may have been making the situation worse. If she related to the private duty nurses in a condescending or suspicious manner, she may have caused them to be more secretive and defensive. If she had approached this last private duty nurse as a colleague whom she respected, she may have had more cooperation.

The nursing supervisor knew Mrs. Schwartz primarily from the information on her hospital admission sheet, daily reports of vital signs and comments from Sally's reports. She seemed to have typecast the patient and blamed her problems on her religion, calling her a "Jewish prima donna." Her apparent prejudice against Jewish women affected her ability to care properly for the patient as a person.

Cultural Values. Mr. Schwartz lived within a professional milieu which requires socializing to attain status. Mrs. Schwartz could no longer meet those needs. She was no longer able to attend social functions with him. She no longer represented beauty and youth to him or his associates. She was dying.

Many men think a woman who has had a hysterectomy can no longer function as a woman. This may have been true of Mr. Schwartz since Mrs. Schwartz claimed that he treated her coolly and would not get close to her after her first surgery.

The Schwartzes' Jewish culture may have shaped some of their values and behavior. They may have experienced prejudice and persecution in their earlier years. If they were immigrants after World War 2, they might have lost everything and everyone close to them. After years of struggle and deprivation, they might need to be in control and want the best. In this case, Mr. Schwartz might have seen "the best" as private duty nurses.

Interpersonal Communications. Whenever emotions, prejudices and values are stirred up, interpersonal communications become hampered. Anger, fear and anxiety on the part of the Schwartzes prevented them from honestly and clearly expressing their needs. The hospital personnel were also angry, hence they were not as sensitive to the patient's needs as they could have been. Sally reported her distrust of the private duty nurse to the supervisor with an emotional overlay of exasperation. Although she had facts to substantiate her suspicions, she had not assembled them adequately before approaching the supervisor. Sally verbalized her frustrations to the supervisor, which may have made her feel better temporarily, but she had not communicated enough evidence of a problem to bring about change. Sally's open distrust of the private duty nurse was most likely preventing open communication at report time. The entire ethical dilemma might have been avoided if all persons involved had been communicating with one another clearly and openly.

Step II: Defining the Problem
In the process of trying to clarify the personal context of the dilemma it may seem as though all we have done is to stir the mud. With so many

factors affecting the situation we have to ask ourselves, Just what is the problem? In order to determine the heart of the problem we need to know three things: (1) who is involved? (2) what issues are at stake? and (3) what further information is needed?

Who Is Involved? We have already looked at the people who are primarily involved when we considered the personal context of the situation, but let's look at them more closely. First, there is Sally. She is in a dilemma primarily because of her unique role as charge nurse. She is responsible *for* and *to* the patient. She is expected to follow physicians' orders, hospital policy and her own conscience. Ultimately she is responsible to God. She is responsible for the care provided by the private duty nurse on her unit, yet she does not feel that she can trust the nurse to give adequate care. At this point some of her responsibilities conflict.

Physicians are also involved in this dilemma. Primarily involved is the doctor who ordered the morphine and gave the verbal order to leave the Levine tube unclamped. We can also assume there are other physicians who are not actively involved, but who have taken no measures to stop the euthanasia efforts. If Mrs. Schwartz was transferred from a medical unit, we can assume that an internist or general practitioner admitted her to the hospital and is probably still on her case. House staff physicians must also be aware of what is going on.

Obviously, Mrs. Schwartz is involved; however, we must question whether she is a victim or an accomplice. She has stated that she would rather die than live as an invalid. Should that statement be taken as a request for euthanasia? Even if she were an active partner in the decision to institute procedures to hasten death, does the desire to die make euthanasia permissible?

Mr. Schwartz has also voiced strongly that his wife should be given "something that will take her out of her misery permanently." The physician told Sally that he was acting on the family's desire to let Mrs. Schwartz die in peace. Apparently Mr. Schwartz has been a definite force in shaping the physician's decision. We have also seen that Mr. Schwartz is a picture of ambivalence and emotional turmoil. He may be faced with overwhelming guilt when his wife dies. He might become suicidal, or he might place all the blame for her death on the doctor, nurses and hospital, and sue them all.

The nursing supervisor is involved although she has refused to intervene at this time. She is responsible for the care given under her supervision. She needs more information to adequately do her job.

The private duty nurse who gave the morphine and left the Levine tube unclamped is directly involved. She has followed doctor's orders, but not in a legal manner. Verbal orders must be written on the chart and signed by the physician before they are legal. She could become a scapegoat in a lawsuit and bear the brunt of the punishment.

Ultimately, other terminal patients could be involved if Mrs. Schwartz's case should set a precedent for active euthanasia in this hospital.

What Issues Are at Stake? Three basic areas outline the issues at stake here: (1) the sanctity of life, (2) respect for civil law, and (3) patients' rights and nurses' responsibilities.

What Further Information Is Needed? We must look at *facts* to clarify these issues. Numerous disciplines provide background knowledge and specific information so that the issues can be more clearly defined.

1. *Biological*—Mrs. Schwartz is in a terminal stage of illness, but the effects of dehydration from fluid deprivation and depressed respirations from morphine toxicity are making death imminent.

2. *Psychological*—Mrs. Schwartz is now beginning to deal with emotional problems she has had since her hysterectomy. She is beginning to express fears and examine her values which could enable her to move toward a peaceful death. This process is being hindered by the euthanasia measures. Although Mr. Schwartz has expressed a desire for his wife's mercy killing, his present emotional state is turbulent. He may regret his decision after his wife's death.

3. *Sociological*—Individuals and groups in our society are beginning to campaign for "the right to die." Not only do they insist on the right to refuse heroic measures, but also the right to take active steps to terminate life.[1] The active measures taken toward Mrs. Schwartz's euthanasia could set a precedent for future cases.

4. *Economic*—Hospital care is expensive. There is no question that it would be a tremendous financial savings for Mr. Schwartz if his wife were to die sooner. Economics is a strong influence on decision making in our society, but the ethical question here must be, Can we measure the worth of human life in dollars? The traditional answer has been no, but

some people question that stance today.[2]

5. *Legal*—Active euthanasia is homicide and clearly illegal at this time in our country.[3] The private duty nurse could become the prime target in a lawsuit if Mr. Schwartz should change his sentiments after the death of his wife. Written orders stated that the Levine tube should be clamped for two hours after eating or drinking and that the morphine was to be given p.r.n. The contrary verbal orders were never written on the chart. However, since the physician verified his verbal orders to Sally, he might also be charged with murder. If Sally did not report the suspicious behavior, she could be charged with negligence. The hospital could also be sued.

6. *Historical*—From the fourth century B.C. when the oath of Hippocrates was drawn up, the most nearly absolute value in Western culture has been the sanctity of human life.[4] The goal of health care has been to preserve human life as well as to promote optimum health. Euthanasia has found proponents from time to time, but until recently Christian thinkers have almost universally opposed it. The loss of a Christian consensus in Western culture has contributed to an increasingly serious consideration of euthanasia on utilitarian and quality-of-life grounds.

7. *Philosophical assumptions*—Philosophical assumptions are drawn from basic beliefs and values. We have already seen how the sanctity of human life has been an assumed value in the history of medical ethics. Recently, the assumption that human life is worth preserving simply because it is human life has been challenged from several quarters. Some have voiced a concern for *quality* of life rather than *quantity* of life, others have demanded the *right* to die when life no longer seems meaningful, and some have even claimed the right to determine when others should die (for example, fetuses with Down's syndrome, acephalous infants and suffering adults). In each case, philosophical assumptions are being made.

Mr. Schwartz's personal philosophy seems to be that his convenience and social success are more important than his wife's life. He has decided that her life is no longer worthwhile.

Mrs. Schwartz has stated that her life lost its meaning and purpose after the hysterectomy, and that she would rather die than live as an invalid.

We must consider, however, whether her statements are a matter of her philosophy of life or are emotional reactions to her husband's treating her as though she were already dead. He has abandoned her for another woman. He does not get close to her. He does not share in her world. She is alone and depressed.

The physician is oriented toward cure. When metastatic carcinoma was discovered, he may have already felt defeat. One of his philosophical assumptions may be that if cure cannot be attained, then the sooner the patient's suffering is over, the better it will be.

Unless the sanctity of human life is seen as an absolute value, euthanasia appears as an attractive option. As long as the law continues to defend the sanctity of human life, euthanasia can be prevented and certainly cannot be ordered by a physician for a nurse to perform. However, in a pluralistic society with a wide assortment of philosophical assumptions, we cannot expect the law to remain unchanged forever. Ethics is based on values, so we must continually ask, Whose values?

8. *Nursing standards*—A sampling of nursing codes provides us with a clear picture of nursing standards regarding situations similar to Mrs. Schwartz's:

I will abstain from whatever is deleterious and mischievous, and will not . . . knowingly administer any harmful drug.
Florence Nightingale Pledge

The nurse acts to safeguard the patient when his care and safety are affected by incompetent, unethical, or illegal conduct of any person.
ANA Code for Nurses

Inherent in nursing is respect for life, dignity and rights of man.
1973 ICN Code for Nurses

Steps III and IV: Proposing Alternatives and Evaluating Alternatives

The world is filled with critics who don't like the present system, or don't agree with the way things are being done. They seldom do much to improve the situation. In order to make ethical decision making practical, we have to propose workable alternatives to unethical practices. Each alternative must be examined for its possible effects and feasibility.

The first and most reasonable alternative for Sally would be to report to the nursing supervisor again, documenting her concerns with all the hard data she can compile. The supervisor may accept the new evidence and take action. On the other hand, she may still refuse to do anything about the situation.

If the supervisor does not respond, Sally would be justified in going to the director of nursing with the facts that she has collected. But she risks losing her supervisor's trust. Moreover, the director of nursing may respect the judgment of the supervisor and take no action at all.

Next Sally could approach the hospital's medical director or the chairman of the hospital ethics committee. They might investigate the situation and reprimand the attending physician, or they might attempt to protect him and do nothing. In going to them Sally risks their resenting her interference and asking her to resign.

If Sally called a lawyer, she would likely get helpful advice and support, though at some cost to her, but she would not get immediate action. Pressing charges would only lead to a long involved court case which probably wouldn't be over until after Mrs. Schwartz died.

Calling the local newspaper and telling them what is going on would prompt immediate action. Mrs. Schwartz would probably be spared the euthanasia attempts, but the results would be inflammatory. The hospital's image would be tarnished, the physician would likely be portrayed as an evil villian, and public sentiment would bring the private duty nurse to trial. Readers might grow to fear being admitted to the hospital and become suspicious of their physicians and nurses.

Finally, Sally could do nothing. Life would be much easier. There would be no interpersonal struggles, no hurt feelings, no angry people. Mrs. Schwartz, though, would die of active euthanasia. This is by far the easiest alternative, but it is also the most unethical one, if life is worth preserving and the law is worth obeying.

After facts are collected and emotional factors considered, the ethical dilemma becomes clearer and the possible alternatives may seem obvious, but we must evaluate these alternatives, weighing their possible negative and positive effects in light of God's Word. Although several options are available, none of them is clear-cut. Sally shared her dilemma with her roommates and asked them to pray with her.

As we prayerfully seek to understand God's will, the most important place to turn is the Scriptures. Think back to the issues at stake: (1) the sanctity of life, (2) respect for civil law and (3) patients' rights and nurses' responsibilities. Each issue can be examined in the light of Scripture. After doing our own biblical research, we could begin to consult other Christians about how they would handle this situation. Let's take each issue separately, then consider how they are interrelated.

The Sanctity of Life. First of all, sit back and think about what you know the Bible says regarding life. Probably the most obvious thing is that God created life and said that it was good (Gen. 1). We can also see patterns where human life is very precious to God. He is constantly involved with his people, guiding and protecting them. There are strict prohibitions against murder in the Old Testament. Jesus devoted a major part of his ministry to healing and even raised some people from the dead. He wept when his friend Lazarus died (Jn. 11:35). There is also a clear message that Jesus came to overcome death and give us new life. Thus, in general, the Bible tends to support the sanctity of human life.

Next take a concordance and look up *life* and all the words you can think of that are related to it, both synonyms and antonyms. Some examples would be *breath, health, death, kill* and *grave.* As you begin to study you'll find that the New Testament talks about two different kinds of life, *bios,* which is usually biological life, and *zoe,* which is life as it is lived in relationship to God. In English both Greek words are translated by the word *life,* but you will begin to see that even though the same word is used two different meanings are developing. At this point a Bible dictionary is helpful. Look up the word *life.* You will find more references and a theological discussion of the significance of the different meanings.

When you look up the word *kill* in a concordance you may come across a passage in 2 Samuel 1 which tells of an Amalekite who reported to David that he killed Saul at his request because he was suffering. David responded in anger and had the Amalekite killed. At first glance this passage looks like a perfect argument against euthanasia. We could assume that David's response should be our response. But we have to be careful. First of all, this is a historical account, not a doctrinal statement. There are other things that David did which we would not want to emulate (for example, 2 Sam. 11). We cannot assume everything he did was right. Second, the context of the passage sheds new light on the subject. Throughout David's lifetime he was concerned about protecting Saul's life because he was the Lord's anointed. It was probably *who* the Amalekite killed, rather than *why* he killed, that angered David. A Bible commentary should clarify the significance of historical events and put them in proper context for you. Whenever you find a passage which looks important, but you question whether it can be applied to your situation, look it up in several commentaries.

From the whole of Scripture some clear principles emerge, and, as you put together your findings, you will be able to form a biblical understanding of life and death. Life is shown to be very precious. It is a gift of God and must be lived in relationship to him. Physical and spiritual death are not clearly differentiated. The punishment for leading someone astray spiritually is just as serious as it is for murder (Mt. 18:6). Being angry with one's brother is equated with killing him (Mt. 5:21-22). The Bible seems to define death as being the point at which a person can no longer praise God (Ps. 88; Job 7:21; Is. 38:18-19; Rom. 8:6). The sanctity of life is clearly established throughout the Scriptures. Premeditated killing is punishable by death, except in the case of war or capital punishment, according to Exodus 20 and 21. Jesus reinforced and strengthened the Old Testament laws against murder (Mt. 5:21-22; 19:18).

Although thorough study in the Scriptures provides us with a solid understanding of the meaning and value of life and the evil of murder, we are still left with no specific teaching about killing a person for compassionate reasons. In fact, we are left with some thorny questions. For instance, we have discovered that the lines between physical life and death, and spiritual life and death are not always clear. Life outside of Christ appears not to be life at all. If this is true, and the Christian will go on living after biological death, does euthanasia really matter? Paul's struggle in Philippians 1:21-26 almost makes it appear as a viable option. Romans 14:8 seems to give further support for that possibility. Even so, Paul does not choose to end his earthly life, but continues to see it as service to God. Our particular dilemma here involves a woman who is not a Christian. What implications does this line of thinking hold for her?

Rather than getting bogged down in our own questions at this point, we need to begin consulting other Christians for their ideas and experience. We have already observed earlier that the Christian church revolutionized health care by not allowing the crippled, blind and unwanted to be killed or left to die. Human life has been held sacred, and apart from the possible exceptions of war and capital punishment, God alone has held the right to decide when a person should die. Denominational statements can provide current perspectives of the church on the issues at stake. In reading publications from my own denominations and several others, I found a lot more questions raised, but no absolute answers, about prolonging life in the face of terminal illness and extreme suffering.[5] Most concentrated on case studies where the definition of death was in question (for example, the need for heroic measures and when to remove a respirator) and seemed to assume that active euthanasia was out of the question.

As we turn to theologians for insight we can expect a great variance of opinion. We can learn as much, however, from the way they reach their conclusions as we can from the conclusions themselves. Joseph Fletcher defends active euthanasia. He takes the ten most common arguments against it and attempts to discredit each.[6] He argues that the issue is not life or death, but the kind of death a person must experience. "Shall we meet death," he asks, "in personal integrity or in personal disintegration? . . . Should there be a moral or a demoralized end to mortal life?"[7] We must deal with his questions even if we do not agree with his position. Helmut Thielicke, while struggling with the question of when to stop attempts to prolong life when all evidence of consciousness is gone, comes out strongly against active euthanasia for the conscious patient. He states that suffering can be an ethical act and even a positive duty, concluding, "Only what is notoriously without meaning can be abandoned to destruction."[8]

So far we have covered the major sources of authority in ethical behavior, but we still do not have an absolute answer to whether it is ethically permissible for Mrs. Schwartz to die because of active measures by the physician and private duty nurse. Yet you probably have some fairly strong leanings. As you begin to sift the information you have collected and apply it to this situation, you could talk it over with a more mature nurse, someone who has experienced similar difficulties. You could also share your findings with a Bible study and prayer group. Perhaps you could discuss some of the problem Bible passages and get their ideas about how they apply to this specific situation. For a Christian patient's view on how it feels to be dying, you could read *Living with Cancer* by Mary Beth Mosler (Chicago: Moody Press, 1979). C. Everett Koop, a Christian physician, presents his views about euthanasia in *The Right to Live; The Right to Die* (Wheaton, IL: Tyndale, 1976).

Respect for Civil Law. Euthanasia is against the law.[9] Some states have formulated legislation to allow patients to refuse heroic life-saving measures, but none permit active euthanasia. So we must consider the Christian's responsibility to uphold the law. Is the Christian bound by the law of the land, or do we answer only to God? Some key words that we might look up are: *law, authority, ruler, king, Caesar, judge, govern, obey, rule, precept, subject, submit.*

One important biblical statement of Christian civil responsibility is found in Romans 13:1-7: "Let every person be subject to the governing authorities. For there is no authority except from God, and those that exist have been instituted by God." This position is fairly consistent throughout Scripture (Tit. 3:1; 1 Pet. 2:13-17; Prov. 8:15; Jn. 19:11), but a gray area begins to develop when we consider Jesus' teaching in Matthew 22:21: "Render therefore to Caesar the things that are Caesar's, and to God the things that are God's." The fine line between what is God's and what is Caesar's is often difficult to draw, especially if we consider that all things belong to God.

In Acts 5:29 Peter and the apostles told the high priest, "We must obey God rather than men." Obeying God in this situation meant preaching the gospel, but could it not also be applied to other ethical dilemmas? Jesus himself broke the accepted interpretation of Jewish law by healing on the sabbath (Jn. 5), by plucking grain for his hungry disciples on the sabbath (Mt. 12), by touching what was declared unclean (Mt. 8:2) and by proclaiming his identity (Mt. 26:61-66). There appears to be a strand in the Scriptures which shows that it is acceptable, even imperative, to break the law when Christian convictions or human compassion are at stake.

If we look at church history for guidelines about obeying the civil authorities, we see a study in contrasts. Under Nero Christians were burned at the stake for practicing their faith. During the Holy Roman

Empire the church and state became so intertwined that the gospel became secondary to politics. During the Reformation Luther preached to the oppressed peasants that they should obey their corrupt rulers, while the Anabaptists attempted to set up alternative communities. Today we can see both extreme positions in the churches in Communist countries. Some obey the law, register with the state and adapt in order to exist in the open. Others meet secretly, disobey and law as it restricts their freedom to worship and evangelize, and refuse to compromise.

A survey of theologians shows a similar divergence of views. For a good summary of the issues at stake from both extremes, see *Morality, Law and Grace* by J. N. D. Anderson (Downers Grove, Ill.: IVP, 1972).

Patients' Rights and Nurses' Responsibilities. In thinking through Scriptural principles relevant to patients' rights and nurses' responsibilities, we would want to give attention to such words as *rights, responsibility, leader, shepherd, sheep, needy, sick, oppressed, afflicted, serve, care, love, neighbor, protect, help, nurse.* The Bible consistently stresses the responsibility of God's people to care faithfully for other people. The poor, the sick and the disadvantaged warrant special attention. God particularly judges persons in positions of responsibility who do not protect and nurture those in their care (Ezek. 34; Jer. 5:30-31; 6:13-15; 12:10-11; 23:1-6). Leaders, a category under which nurses may fall, are compared to shepherds. One responsibility of shepherds is to protect their flocks from life-threatening danger. Jesus equates service and caring for needy people with caring for him in Matthew 25. Jesus also commanded us to love our neighbors as ourselves (Mt. 22:39). Love for others involves desiring and working toward the best good for them. Love includes a willingness to empathize with people and to protect them from evil (Rom. 12:9-21).

Church history has shown practical applications of the Christian's responsibility to protect the rights of others. Nursing orders and hospitals were established during the Crusades. Homes for the poor and for orphans, as well as hospitals, were established and maintained by churches in this country before the government became the primary provider of welfare services. Care of the sick, the poor, the disadvantaged and the oppressed has been a priority of the church throughout its history, in spite of its blindness to the needs of many persons over the years.

The writings of contemporary Christians abound on the subject of caring for others. Francis Schaeffer reminds us that love is the "mark of the Christian."[10] David Augsburger insists that love involves "caring enough to confront."[11] Dosia Carlson, a patient, cries out to be cared for as a person with rights and feelings.[12]

Step V: Developing a Plan of Action

The data we have collected thus far can be staggering and confusing. Before a specific plan of action can be developed, all of our information must be sifted, compared, related and evaluated. We need to look at the biblical material in the light of the facts about the dilemma. Mrs. Schwartz is a person whose life is precious. She has rights and feelings. She said her life is not worth living as an invalid, and her husband, physician and private duty nurse have accepted her statement as a request for euthanasia. She has not been given the opportunity by anyone except, perhaps, Sally to explain the meaning of her statement or to express her psychological and spiritual needs. Her rights as a human being are being violated and the sanctity of her life is not being respected. The law in this case is protecting her right to life. It should be upheld. Sally is committed to Mrs. Schwartz as a person in her care. As a Christian who is a shepherd and as a charge nurse who is responsible for all patients on her unit, Sally must protect Mrs. Schwartz from harm.

Sally herself has no power to actually change the situation. The private duty nurse has been hired by the patient with hospital approval. Sally cannot remove her from the case. Neither can Sally prevent the physician's orders from being carried out since she does not provide direct care. The supervisor, however, has the power to remove the private duty nurse from the case by withdrawing her acceptance in the registry. She has no control over the physician, but it would be appropriate for her to inform the chief of surgery about his activities. He, in turn, could inform the staff physicians who could then vote to either reprimand the surgeon or remove him from the hospital staff.

As Sally moves into action she will need continued prayer support and encouragement from other Christians. Confrontation is painful and energy-sapping. It can cause a person to feel alone and afraid. The support of the Christian community will help to reinforce the presence of

God with Sally as she acts on her convictions.

Sally will also need to re-examine her motives and attitudes before she acts. We have already noted that her own prejudice against private duty nurses has hindered communication. She will have to take care that her zeal to protect Mrs. Schwartz does not become a vendetta against the nurse.

Sally has already confronted the persons directly involved, the physician and the private duty nurse, but she will have to evaluate whether she has communicated enough information to them and actually owned her opinions before she reports them to higher authorities. Perhaps she could be more specific about her concerns: (1) that the patient will die as a direct result of the morphine and dehydration, (2) that she may not be ready to die, even though she said that her life was not worth living, (3) that her husband may regret his decision later and suffer extreme psychological distress, (4) that euthanasia is illegal, (5) that the sanctity of Mrs. Schwartz's life is being violated and (6) that her rights as a human being are at stake.

As Sally prepares to go through the proper channels to change the situation, she must be ready to offer the documentation that the supervisor requested earlier. The facts should be in writing, making Sally accountable for what she reports.

In the actual case from which this study was drawn, Sally reported the situation again to her supervisor, supporting her position with adequate facts. The nursing supervisor saw the seriousness of the situation immediately and took action. The private duty nurse was removed from the case and warned that she would be removed from the registry if she repeated her mistakes. The supervisor spoke with the physician, asked him if her information was accurate and, when assured that it was, told him that she would report him to the medical ethics committee and the chief of staff if he did not change his method of treatment. He complied.

With no more private duty nurses available, Mrs. Schwartz was forced to receive care from the usual floor personnel. Sally spent extra time helping her to verbalize her fears and frustrations, and at Mrs. Schwartz's request she prayed with her. Mrs. Schwartz visibly relaxed and became much more peaceful. She died four weeks later.

Part Two
Clinical
Case
Studies

Introduction

Ethics is hard work. Ethical decision making takes time if it is done well. Often in the middle of an ethical dilemma there is little time to go home and do in-depth Bible study, then to go to the library and thoroughly research the issues at stake. One way you can avoid giving in to instinct and emotion for ethical direction is to be prepared in advance.

Part two is designed with this in mind—helping you to prepare in advance for a wide variety of ethical decisions. In a preliminary study (pp. 96-98) you are encouraged to think through your own philosophy of nursing. Eight case studies from actual clinical experience follow (pp. 100-128), each representative of others which have happened elsewhere and which may well happen to you. (Names and places have been changed to protect the persons involved.)

These case studies are designed to be used as individual preparation for the series of small group discussions which follow (pp. 129-30), though they can stand on their own if you do not have a group with which to share. Keep in mind, though, that consulting other Christians is an important step in the decision-making process.

For each case study, read through the situation and then work through the whole decision-making process as though you were the nurse involved. Directions and suggested resources follow each case. The resources are not exhaustive, but should start you thinking. Be sure to carry the process through to developing a plan of action. The more you try to put yourself in the shoes of the nurse involved, the more productive your study will be.

When you are finished you still won't have any easy answers—each dilemma carries with it its own frustrations and heartaches—but you will be better prepared to evaluate objectively your own dilemmas and to move toward responsible action.

Preliminary Study:
A Christian Philosophy of Nursing

Moral values and ethical conduct spring from inner convictions and a personal philosophy of life. In particular, our ethics as nurses will reflect our philosophy of nursing. To help you sharpen your philosophy of nursing read through the following statement developed by members of the Nurses Christian Fellowship and then answer the questions which follow.

We believe each person is created to be an integrated whole—a biological, psychosocial and spiritual being. We believe each person can attain and maintain wholeness as an individual when these dimensions are cared for and/or restored.

We believe the nurse, as a vital "change agent," is involved as a member of the health team in restoring and/or maintaining wholeness during times of health, illness or dying. We, therefore, believe the nurse should be actively involved in restoring and maintaining the spiritual wholeness of patients as well as ministering to their physical and psychosocial needs. We further believe that the degree of spiritual wholeness in the nurse will determine her/his interest and ability to clearly identify and meet these needs.

We believe spiritual wholeness begins as an individual is brought into a vital relationship to God through faith in Jesus Christ. This relationship is an ever-increasing and maturing trust-relationship between the restored individual and God.

We believe the nurse who is experiencing a dynamically restored relationship with God through Jesus Christ, that is the Christian nurse, is developing a trust-relationship with him from which issues unselfish love and concern for self and others. This enhances the nurse's resources and potential ability to give compassionate, sensitive, thorough care to patients and their families.

We believe the Christian nurse has the potential to recognize that God is present and powerful in each situation and sees in it an opportunity to please and communicate Jesus Christ. We believe that given guidelines and assistance in assessing and meeting spiritual needs, the nurse will be able to recognize a patient's spiritual needs and assist in meeting these needs through personal intervention and referral. Recognizing God's presence and power enables the nurse to demonstrate stability and convey confidence while responding to human need and fulfilling professional obligations with the attitude of serving God and others.

We believe the Christian nurse who understands herself/himself in relationship to God will have a worldwide concern for client-centered nursing and will participate responsibly in planning, developing and upholding the standards of nursing education and practice. We believe the Christian nurse will be continually increasing in personal development and professional competency, conscientiously serving supervisors, peers and subordinates.

Finally, we believe that the Christian nurse, motivated by a personal relationship with God will function in accord with principles revealed by God in the Bible and to assist "the individual (and family), sick or well, in the performance of those activities contributing to health or its recovery (or to a peaceful death) that would be performed unaided if he had the necessary strength, will or knowledge, and to do this in such a way as to help him gain independence as rapidly as possible" (Virginia Henderson, The Nature of Nursing [New York: Macmillan, 1966], p. 15).

(This statement is adapted from "This We Believe: A Christian Philosophy of Nursing," developed by Nurses Christian Fellowship Ad Hoc Committee, 1968-69, revised 1976.)

Study Questions

1. Do you agree with the first paragraph's definition of personhood? Does this agree with what you learned in nursing school?

2. How does the second paragraph characterize the role of the nurse? Do you see yourself in this role? Do you believe that these are essential nursing functions? Why or why not?

3. According to the third paragraph, how do we obtain spiritual health? What is the significance of describing this relationship as "an ever-increasing and maturing trust-relationship between the restored individual and God"?

4. How does the fourth paragraph define a Christian nurse? How does a Christian nurse differ from other nurses?

5. What is the Christian nurse's source of power? Is it ethical to meet spiritual needs of patients? Why or why not? What does the fifth paragraph suggest is the nurse's realm of responsibility and influence?

6. What can nurses do to uphold standards of nursing practice and education? How are ethics and competency related? How is "conscientiously serving supervisors, peer and subordinates" related to nursing ethics?

7. Does your definition of nursing agree with Henderson's quoted in the last paragraph? If not, write out a definition of your own. How has your relationship with God affected the way you practiced nursing over the past week? (Think of specific examples.)

(These questions are adapted from "Christian Perspectives on Nursing," a series of seminars developed by Judy Van Heukelem and Lynn Ellis for nursing students at the Univ. of California Medical Center in San Francisco.)

Steps I—IV.A of the Ethical Decision-Making Process

The questions below are designed to help you work through Steps I through IV.A of the decision-making process for each of the case studies which follow.

Step I. Clarifying the Personal Context
A. What is the emotional climate?
B. What personal biases are evident?
C. What cultural values are involved?
D. What communication problems exist?

Step II. Defining the Problem
A. Who is involved?
B. What issues are at stake?
C. Gathering further information:
   1. What biological facts are relevant (including medicine, genetics, ecology)?
   2. What psychological problems are evident?
   3. What sociological factors are involved?
   4. What economic factors enter into the dilemma? How?
   5. What laws and policies are relevant?
   6. What light does history shed on the problem?
   7. What underlying philosophies shape people's attitudes?
   8. What nursing standards or codes are being violated?

Step III. Proposing Alternatives
What are several alternative courses of action?

Step IV. Evaluating Alternatives
A. What are the probable effects and general feasibility of each alternative?

Case Study A: When Values Clash

Joy Gardner was a student in her Maternal-Child Health experience when she was assigned to Labor and Delivery. She arrived on the floor excited about the possibility of seeing her first delivery.

"This is 'T.A. Day,'" the head nurse told her. "You can take Susie Smith over there."

As she looked over at the thirteen-year-old girl to whom she was assigned, Joy was confused. "Why are they doing tonsillectomies in the delivery room?" she asked the head nurse.

"Not tonsillectomies, Sweetie—abortions. We try to schedule them all on the same day," she responded, then turned and went into another patient's room.

Joy's heart sank. Abortions! She was sure she was against them. She had long ago decided that she would never have one herself, but what about caring for women who were having them?

Susie was dressing a Barbie doll as Joy went into the room. "You're going to have an abortion this morning?" Joy said.

"Yeah, I guess so," Susie answered not looking up from the doll.

"How did you come to that decision?" Joy asked.

"My Mom said they'd kick me out of school if I was pregnant. I don't really care about school, but I'd miss my friends. Besides I've had this done once before, and it don't really hurt too bad. I guess having a baby would hurt a lot more."

Joy's head was full of questions she wanted to ask Susie, but she didn't know how or where to begin. "I'll be back in a few minutes," she told her as she headed out to the nurses' station to talk to anyone who would listen.

The head nurse was sitting at the desk, working on a chart. "This is Susie's second abortion," Joy began. "She acts like it's nothing! Who's to say that she won't just go right back out and get pregnant again? Doesn't she know that's a baby in there? All she's thinking about is herself and how to avoid pain and hassles. Has anyone told her about the seriousness of what she's doing?"

The head nurse chuckled, "We aren't here to moralize, Honey. We only take care of patients. If they need nursing care, we nurse them. It doesn't matter if they happen to be a streetwalker or the pope."

Joy's instructor appeared as the conversation ended.

"Your little gal here seems to have some problems with her assignment today," the head nurse said to the instructor as she walked away carrying the chart.

"What seems to be the problem, Joy?" the instructor asked.

"I just don't think I can take care of abortion patients! My patient is a thirteen-year-old girl having her second abortion. I just can't participate in that. I believe abortion is murder. I don't want to be a murderer!" Joy was in tears when she finished.

"Well, you can go home if you'd like," the instructor began. "Of course, I'll have to give you a failing grade for today's clinical. Abortion patients have just as many needs as anyone else, you know, maybe more. You can't just cop out on them."

Joy did not know what to do. Susie obviously had needs, but Joy wasn't sure she could meet them. She wanted to talk to her about the seriousness of what she was doing, but that could really cause problems. It might cause pathological guilt if Susie went ahead with the abortion. If she decided not to have the abortion, Susie's mother, the nursing staff, the doctor and probably a lot of other people would be upset with Joy. She thought maybe the instructor was right—going home would be copping out. But what else could she do? ■

Two major issues come into focus in this situation. First is the question of whether or not abortion is murder. Is it killing a human person? Can a Christian assent to the practice? Second, Joy was faced with the problem of whether or not caring for Susie would be condoning her actions. What does the Bible say about caring for someone whose values conflict with ours?

Steps I—IV.A

Turn to page 99 and answer the questions there in relation to this case study.

Step IV Continued

To complete your evaluation of alternatives answer the questions below, taking into account relevant Scripture and other reading. Remember the Scripture and readings suggested are not exhaustive. A concordance and Bible dictionary can provide further resources.

Life before Birth:

1. When does human life begin?

Eccles. 11:5	Lk. 1:15	Lk. 1:41-44
Gal. 1:15	Eph. 1:4-5	

2. How does God view fetal life?

Ex. 21:22-25	Ps. 139:13-16	Is. 49:1
Is. 49:5	Jer. 1:5	

Other Reading:

The Exodus 21:22-25 passage is controversial. Some scholars have argued that this passage sees the fetus as less than human in calling for a monetary payment in the event of a miscarriage—that is, a spontaneous abortion or stillbirth. Others have argued that the qualification "yet no harm follows" explicitly limits the idea of miscarriage to a premature, live and healthy birth. The death of the fetus or any injury to it would call for corresponding punishment—"life for life, eye for eye, . . ." Thus the passage teaches the full humanity of the fetus. See:

Jack W. Cottrell, "Abortion and the Mosaic Law," *Christianity Today* (March 16, 1973), pp. 6-9.

R. Alan Cole, *Exodus* (IVP, 1973), p. 169.

The sanctity of human life is at stake here too. See chapter seven for a discussion of the biblical and theological background. See also:

Norman Anderson, *Issues of Life and Death* (IVP, 1976), pp. 11-33, 58-84.

Clifford Bajema, *Abortion and the Meaning of Personhood* (Baker, 1974).

Christian Medical Society, *Birth Control and the Christian* (Tyndale, 1969).

C. Everett Koop, *The Right to Live; The Right to Die* (Tyndale, 1976), pp. 23-80.

John T. Noonan, *The Morality of Abortion* (Harvard Univ. Press, 1970).

Eldon Weisheit, *Abortion? Resources for Pastoral Counseling* (Concordia, 1976).

Caring for Someone Who Has Different Values:

1. How did Jesus relate to people with values different from his?

Mt. 9:10-13	Mk. 10:17-22	Lk. 23:39-43
Jn. 4:7-30	Jn. 8:3-11	

2. What principles are given in Scripture about caring for other people?

Is. 58:6-12	Mt. 22:37-40	Mt. 25:31-46
Lk. 10:25-37	Rom. 12:9-21	

Other Reading:

Rebecca Manley Pippert, *Out of the Saltshaker* (IVP, 1979).

Kenneth F. W. Prior, *The Gospel in a Pagan Society* (IVP, 1975).

Elizabeth Skoglund, *Where Do I Go to Buy Happiness?* (IVP, 1972), pp. 99-117.

Step V

Now write a plan of action as though you were in Joy's place.

Case Study B: When Rights, Responsibilities and Orders Conflict

Connie Evans began her first nursing position on a medical unit in a large city hospital. After she had been there about six months, just as she was gaining confidence in her nursing abilities, she refused to give an ordered dose of morphine she felt was unsafe. The director of nursing, under pressure from the medical staff, asked Connie to resign because of the incident.

Connie felt her actions were justified and appropriate. The patient, Mrs. Johnson, had terminal cancer. She had been on smaller doses of morphine which seemed to control her pain well; however, her respirations were becoming depressed. During the past two days Mrs. Johnson had begun to talk about death. She told her family the hymns she wanted sung at her funeral and mentioned that she was looking forward to seeing Jesus and her husband, who had died previously. Her son and daughter became anxious whenever Mrs. Johnson began to talk about death. They requested a conference with the attending physician. After talking with the family and checking Mrs. Johnson, the attending physician doubled Mrs. Johnson's morphine dosage and increased its frequency. He handed Connie the chart after writing the order and said, "Here, I want this to begin *now*."

Connie was shocked. She considered Mrs. Johnson's talk of death to be a positive growth experience for her and her family, even though it made the family uncomfortable. She had encouraged Mrs. Johnson to verbalize her feelings about death and was attempting to support the son and daughter in the process. The increased dosage of morphine would mean imminent and, most likely, premature death.

As Connie stood holding the chart, trying to decide what to do, the physician roared, "I said give it to her now!"

"Her respirations are only six per minute," Connie replied. "It might kill her."

"Young lady," the physician answered, as he squinted at Connie's name tag and wrote her name on a slip of paper, "I've been on the staff here for twenty-eight years, and the custom has always been that I write the orders and the nurses carry them out. Are you going to give that morphine, or do I have to call your supervisor?"

"I don't believe it's safe, Dr. Jones. I can't give it," Connie replied. "Would you like me to page the supervisor?"

Dr. Jones paged the nursing supervisor and poured out his anger over what he called Connie's "insubordination." Connie was called to the nursing office about an hour later and told that she would be reduced in status to an aide. She felt strongly that a Christian should be submissive to authority, so she decided to accept the situation and trust God to vindicate her for doing what she felt was right. A week later Connie was asked to resign by the director of nursing, who stated that the chief of staff had demanded the resignation after a medical staff meeting. ■

In this situation we are again faced with a dilemma involving the sanctity of life. Connie was torn between what she perceived as her right to refuse to give what she believed to be an unsafe medication in order to protect a patient's life and her responsibility to carry out the physician's order. Her responsibility to the patient came in conflict with her responsibility to the physician.

Steps I—IV.A
Turn to page 99 and answer the questions there in relation to this case study.

Step IV Continued
To complete your evaluation of alternatives answer the questions below, taking into account relevant Scripture and other reading. Remember the Scripture and readings suggested here are not exhaustive. A concordance and Bible dictionary can provide further resources.

The Sanctity of Life:
Review chapter eight.

Responsibility to Persons in Our Care:

1. The Bible uses the concept of a shepherd (among others) as a model for persons in positions of responsibility. What are the duties of a shepherd?

Ezek. 34:1-16   1 Pet. 5:1-3

2. How does Jesus view nursing care?

Mt. 25:31-46   Lk. 10:25-37

3. How does God view our unwillingness to carry out our responsibility to those with whom we have been entrusted?

Jer. 5:30-31   Jer. 6:13-15   Jer. 12:10-17

Jer. 23:1-6

Other Reading:

Irene L. Beland and Joyce Y. Passos, *Clinical Nursing* (Macmillan, 1975), pp. 3-12.

Leah Curtin, *The Mask of Euthanasia* (N.C.F.L., Inc., 1976), pp. 31-33.

Laurel Archer Copp, "Nursing As Ministry," *Ethical Issues in Nursing* (Catholic Hospital Association, 1976), pp. 65-70.

Responsibility to Persons in Authority:

1. What should our attitude be toward persons in authority?

Eph. 6:5-8   1 Tim. 2:1-2   1 Tim. 6:1-2

1 Pet. 2:13-17   1 Pet. 5:5-7

2. To what extent must we obey authority?

Acts 5:29   Rom. 13:1-7   Rev. 13:1—14:12

Other Reading:

Michael Green, *New Life, New Lifestyle* (IVP, 1973), pp. 119-21.

David Field, *Taking Sides* (IVP, 1975), pp. 82-102.

Step V

Now write a plan of action as though you were in Connie's place.

Case Study C:
When the Truth Hurts

Chris began giving evening care late. She was a bit flustered. Most of the postoperative patients had returned on her shift so that all she had had time to do was to pass out medicines and make rounds on the post-ops every fifteen minutes. As she rubbed Mr. Adkins's back he asked, "Nurse, what was that blue and white capsule I got tonight? I've never had that one before." Chris couldn't remember, so she told him that she would check and let him know. In the meantime she moved on to get the next patient ready for bed.

The next patient was Mr. Duska. He didn't have any lotion. Chris checked the floor supply. No lotion. She grabbed a medicine cup and ducked into Mr. Adkins's room, "May I borrow some of your lotion for someone who doesn't have any?" Mr. Adkins agreed and asked if Chris had checked on his new capsule. "No, I haven't had a chance, yet," Chris replied. "Thanks for the lotion." She returned to Mr. Duska and set the lotion on the bedside table as she helped him turn to his side. The phone at the desk rang. Chris ran to answer it.

"This is the admissions office. We have an admission for you. He'll be coming up from the emergency room. The diagnosis is possible appendicitis." Chris was beginning to panic. She quickly got a chart ready, then ran back to Mr. Duska, hoping to finish his P.M. care before the emergency room called to report on the admission.

"Whew! They sure did change the flavor of that Maalox!" Mr. Duska commented as Chris entered his room.

"Maalox? What Maalox? I didn't give you any Maalox," Chris answered.

"Yes you did, you left it beside my bed. I figured you didn't have time to tell me about it in all the rush."

Chris felt her stomach hardening into a sickening knot. She rubbed Mr. Duska's back using the talcum powder in his drawer and thought over what she would do next. She realized that she'd have to fill out an incident report. She wondered what effect the back lotion would have on Mr. Duska and whether it would be harmful. Part of her question was answered when suddenly he asked for a bedpan. She decided that she'd better call the intern right away. As she went out to call she remembered Mr. Adkins's blue and white capsule, so she checked his Kardex. No, he didn't have anything of that description ordered, but his roommate was on Lincocin. That meant his roommate probably did not get his Lincocin. Christ felt the tears welling up in her eyes.

The emergency room called to report on the new admission as the patient arrived by stretcher at the nurses' station. Chris got caught up in the rush of admitting the patient, transcribing orders onto the Kardex, and answering requests for sleep and pain medications. She put off calling the intern. She took a Lincocin capsule to Mr. Adkins's roommate. It was three hours late, but at least he got it.

Finally the excitement waned, and Chris sat down at the nurses' station. She picked up the phone and dialed the intern's number, pulling out two incident report forms from the file drawer as she waited for him to answer. She reported about Mr. Duska drinking the back lotion which made the intern laugh heartily, "He'll be fine—he probably needed a little laxative anyhow!"

Then she reported Mr. Adkins getting the Lincocin. "Is he allergic to it or anything?" the intern asked. Assured that he wasn't and that he had had no ill effects, the intern told Chris to take a verbal order for one dose of Lincocin to cover the error.

"No, that's okay, I'd rather not do that," Chris said, her conscience beginning to hurt. She hung up and began to think. She had only planned to fill out two incident reports, but what about the patient who had gotten his Lincocin three hours late? It was ordered to be given every six hours. He'd be getting another dose in three hours. It probably wouldn't do any harm. After all, he had gotten it—the dose hadn't been skipped entirely. The hospital had a policy that R.N.'s who accumulated three medicine error incident reports in their files had to take the L.P.N. pharmacology course before they could be assigned to medicines again. This would make three med errors in one night. Chris sat, staring at the file drawer, struggling to decide if she should fill out the third incident report. ■

Just how important is it for a Christian to tell the whole truth? Are little cover-ups permissible? Chris felt it was important to save her reputation. She did not want to be humiliated.

Steps I—IV.A
Turn to page 99 and answer the questions there in relation to this case study.

Step IV Continued
To complete your evaluation of alternatives answer the questions below, taking into account relevant Scripture and other reading. Remember the Scripture and readings suggested here are not exhaustive. A concordance and Bible dictionary can provide further resources.

Truth-telling:

1. What is the importance of telling the truth in human relationships?

Ex. 20:16   Deut. 5:20   Eph. 4:25

2. What are God's standards for truth-telling?

Ps. 51:6-14   Is. 59:14-20   Jn. 14:6

Other Reading:

Michael Green, *New Life, New Lifestyle* (IVP, 1973), pp. 119-21.

Geri Rush, "God's Ethics," *The Nurses Lamp* (Nov. 1974), p. 2.

Professional Conduct:

1. What is the importance of a Christian's professional reputation?

Lk. 6:26   1 Cor. 10:32-33   2 Cor. 6:3-10

1 Thess. 1:10-12   1 Pet. 2:11-12

2. What attitudes should characterize our professional lives?

Eph. 4:1-3   Phil. 2:3-8   Col. 3:12-15

1 Pet. 5:6-7

3. How does God use apparent dishonor in the lives of his people?

2 Cor. 4:7-18   2 Cor. 7:9-10   Phil. 1:12-14

1 Pet. 1:3-7   1 Pet. 5:8-10

Other Reading:
   David Field, *Taking Sides* (IVP, 1975), pp. 82-102.
   Michael Green, *New Life, New Lifestyle* (IVP, 1973), pp. 104-5.

Step V
Now write a plan of action as though you were in Chris's place.

Case Study D:
When Two Good
Purposes Conflict

Tom Sanders was admitted to ICU after spending most of the night in the operating room. He had been stabbed fifteen times in the chest during a gang fight. Surgeons had attempted to repair his punctured heart and lungs, but his prognosis was hopeless. He lay comatose, connected to a respirator, chest tubes, a cardiac monitor, IVs and a Foley catheter. By noon his EEG was flat.

Tom was the youngest of eight children. An older brother had been killed in a gang fight the year before. His family was poor, but proud. They had refused to accept welfare, but they had no hospitalization insurance.

Tom's mother wept softly as Cathy Wilkens, an ICU nurse, sat with her. Cathy was on her way home from work when she saw Mrs. Sanders in the hospital lobby and stopped to talk with her. "He's my baby and he's gonna die. I just know it!" wailed Mrs. Sanders. Cathy swallowed hard. A repeat EEG, completed as she was leaving the unit, had confirmed the diagnosis of brain death. The resident was looking for Mrs. Sanders to ask if Tom's kidneys could be used for transplanting to another patient. All indications showed the kidneys would be a perfect match.

"Mrs. Sanders," Cathy asked gently, "if Tom does die, how would you feel if his kidneys could be used to give someone else life?" Tears flowed from Mrs. Sanders's eyes, "Oh no! I just want my baby buried with all his body together!"

Cathy knew that a power struggle would ensue. The resident was just as determined to get permission to use the kidneys as Mrs. Sanders was to prevent it. She changed the subject, talked for a while and went home.

The next day when Cathy came to work Tom was still on the respirator. Another EEG had been performed. It showed no brain activity. The family had not been told. They were still refusing to sign a release for Tom's kidneys. The resident was planning to keep Tom on the respirator until they agreed.

Cathy talked with the doctor, suggesting that it was not fair to withhold the truth from Tom's family since it was prolonging their grief and substantially increasing their expenses. Each day in ICU was adding thousands of dollars to their bill, although Tom was already legally dead.

The resident became indignant, "There is a man on nephrology who needs a transplant now. One of this man's kidneys could save his life."

"Can't you at least tell Tom's family that he is dead?" Cathy pleaded.

"Not until they sign a release for his kidneys," the doctor retorted.

Cathy struggled with her conscience. Should she take the risk of telling the family herself? Instead she decided to explain the urgent need for the kidney. After trying without success, she hated herself for playing along with the resident's scheme, but did not have the courage to do otherwise.

"He's dead, isn't he?" Tom's mother asked.

"His heart is still beating," Cathy replied.

"He'll never get better," Mrs. Sanders said knowingly. ■

Cathy was in an awkward position. She felt that in order to maintain a good working relationship with the resident she would have to deny Tom's family their right to know about his brain death. The resident had a good point—Tom's kidneys could save someone else's life. But the decision was not his to make. Here we have a situation where the Bible has no clear-cut answer. Several biblical principles seem to be in conflict. Some principles must be violated if others are followed.

Steps I—IV.A
Turn to page 99 and answer the questions there in relation to this case study.
Step IV Continued
To complete your evaluation of alternatives answer the questions below, taking into account relevant Scripture and other reading. Remember the Scripture and readings suggested here are not exhaustive. A concor-

dance and Bible dictionary can provide further resources.

Withholding the Truth:

1. Review Case Study C, "When the Truth Hurts."

2. What is our responsibility when we know someone else is not telling the truth?

Ex. 23:1 Eph. 5:6-17

Other Reading:

Joseph Fletcher, *Morals and Medicine* (Beacon, 1954), pp. 3-64.

Paul Ramsey, *The Patient As Person* (Yale Univ. Press, 1970), pp. 5-40.

Respect for the Body:

1. What is the Christian view of the body after death?

1 Cor. 15:35-44 Phil. 3:20-21

2. How does the removal or destruction of body parts affect a person's afterlife? In other words, does donating body parts violate Christian principles?

Mk. 9:43-48 2 Cor. 5:1

3. What importance does the Bible place on proper burial?

Gen. 23:19-20 Gen. 25:8-9 Gen. 49:29-33

Mt. 26:10-13 Mk. 15:45—16:1 Acts 5:5-6

Acts 5:10 Acts 8:2

Other Reading:

James B. Nelson, *Rediscovering the Person in Medical Care* (Augsburg, 1976), pp. 15-31.

Paul Ramsey, *The Patient As Person* (Yale Univ. Press, 1970), pp. 198-215.

Stewardship over God's Creation:

1. What all has God entrusted to us? What are the limits of our control?

Gen. 1:26-28 Ps. 8:5-8 Heb. 2:6-9

2. How does God view our management of money, especially other people's?

Lk. 16:10-12

3. What should our attitude as Christians be toward other people's possessions?

Ex. 20:17 Lk. 12:13-21

Other Reading:

Norman Anderson, *Issues of Life and Death* (IVP, 1976), pp. 85-107.

David Field, *Taking Sides* (IVP, 1975), pp. 37-42.

Giving in Love:

1. What should our attitude be toward someone who asks for something we have?

Mt. 5:42-48   Lk. 6:30-31

2. What is the ultimate gift?

Jn. 15:13   Rom. 5:7-8   Eph. 5:2

3. Do we have the right to decide what, or how much, another person should give?

Mt. 7:1-5   Jn. 21:20-22   Rom. 2:1-4

2 Cor. 9:7

Other Reading:

Michael Green, *New Life, New Lifestyle* (IVP, 1973), pp. 81-82.

Helmut Thielicke, *The Doctor As Judge of Who Shall Live and Who Shall Die* (Fortress, 1976), pp. 21-32.

Step V

Now write a plan of action as though you were in Cathy's place.

Case Study E:
When the System
Is Unjust

Joanne Murray wanted a challenge when she graduated from nursing school, so she applied for a position as a staff nurse in a large urban medical center which had a good reputation for its quality nursing care. Several of her friends had been patients at this medical center and had highly recommended it to Joanne. A guided tour of the facilities convinced Joanne that this would be the ideal place to work.

After a week of orientation Joanne was sent to the floor where she would work. Her idealism was quickly shattered. It was a medical unit for patients on welfare. Most of them required total care, yet the ratio of patients to staff was often ten to one on days. On evenings and nights the situation was worse. Other floors with private patients were well staffed. The head nurse was an alcoholic with a foul temper who pitted her staff against one another. The atmosphere was thick with hostility. The average length of stay for personnel was three months.

Joanne was committed to giving good nursing care, yet she found it impossible to provide even adequate care. She became depressed and discouraged and began to wonder if she wanted to stay in nursing at all. She volunteered to work permanent nights to avoid the problems of relating to the day shift, especially the head nurse. One night when things were fairly quiet Joanne confided her frustrations to the night supervisor. The supervisor responded sympathetically, saying, "I know things are bad on three South, but there's nothing we can do about it. Perhaps we could transfer you to another floor. You've served enough time here."

Joanne felt she could not accept the offer with a clear conscience. To go to another floor would not improve nursing care on three South. It would merely remove it from her experience. Joanne was deeply concerned about the patients who were receiving such poor care.

The following week Joanne met the hospital administrator at a church supper. He asked how she liked working at the medical center. She was so caught up in her feelings of frustration that she told him honestly and asked, "Why is the staffing on three South so much worse than on the private floors?"

"Oh, but it's not!" he replied. "We have exactly the same number of nurses on each unit."

"Yes, but the other units have fewer patients, and most of those patients require much less physical care than ours do," Joanne responded.

The administrator hesitated, then said, "Well, we have to provide better care for our paying patients. They are our public relations force. If they don't receive good care, we would be in trouble financially. Then we couldn't provide care for anybody."

Joanne swallowed hard to hold back the tears of anger and frustration. She wondered how Christians could perpetuate such inequality and injustice. Yet she felt powerless. She went home and cried. ■

Most Christians have been taught to submit to authorities and bear with any suffering that ensues. But what if that submission comes into conflict with our responsibility to care for the poor and oppressed? How much influence should economics have on our actions? What should a Christian do about unjust systems? Joanne was faced with all of these questions, but felt helpless in her situation. What could she do that would really help in this situation?

Steps I—IV.A
Turn to page 99 and answer the questions there in relation to this case study.
Step IV Continued
To complete your evaluation of alternatives answer the questions below, taking into account relevant Scripture and other reading. Remember the Scripture and readings suggested here are not exhaustive. A concordance and Bible dictionary can provide further resources.

Economics:
1. What kinds of people was Jesus concerned about in his ministry?

Mk. 1:40-45	Mk. 10:13-16	Mt. 8:5-17
Mt. 11:19	Mt. 21:32	Lk. 7:37-50
Lk. 13:11-13	Lk. 15:1-2	Lk. 19:1-10
Jn. 4:46-54		

2. How did Jesus view the poor?

Lk. 6:20	Mt. 19:21	Mt. 26:11
1 Sam. 2:7-8		

3. What is the biblical view of material wealth?

Jas. 5:16	Jer. 9:23-24	Mt. 19:23-30
2 Cor. 9:6-15	Acts 2:44-45	Ps. 112:1-3
1 Tim. 6:17-19		

Other Reading:

Michael Green, *New Life, New Lifestyle* (IVP, 1973), pp. 81-82.

Harold C. Letts, *Health Care in America: A National Illness* (Lutheran Church in America, Division for Mission in North America, 1974), chapter 4, pp. 43-51, and chapter 9, pp. 103-14.

Justice:
1. What is the biblical view of justice?

Lk. 6:27	Amos 6:1-8	Deut. 16:18-20
Jas. 2:1-13	Mt. 23:23-24	Acts 24:24-25

2. What is our individual responsibility in bringing about justice?

Is. 1:17	Mic. 6:8	Jas. 2:14-17
Jas. 4:17	Ps. 37:27-28	Ps. 82:3-4

Other Reading:

Klaus Bockmuehl, *Evangelicals and Social Ethics* (IVP, 1979), pp. 17-18.

John W. Alexander, *Practical Criticism* (IVP, 1976).

Brian Griffiths, *Is Revolution Change?* (IVP, 1972), chapter 5, pp. 84-105.

Changing the System:
1. Jesus summarizes the effects of his gospel in Luke 4:18-19. What implications does this have for Christian action?
2. What reputation does Jesus have among the Pharisees?

Mt. 22:15-16	Mk. 12:13-14	Lk. 20:19-26

3. How does Jesus handle corruption and injustice?

Mk. 11:15-19   Lk. 11:42-46   Jn. 2:14-16

4. What did Paul do when he saw deceit and corruption?

2 Cor. 11:12-15   Eph. 5:6-13   2 Thess. 3:1-2

5. What attitudes should characterize our social action?

Is. 1:16-17   1 Pet. 5:6-11   Lk. 6:27-36

Lk. 12:32-37

Other Reading:

Klaus Bockmuehl, *Evangelicals and Social Ethics* (IVP, 1979), pp. 17-39.

C. René Padilla, *The New Face of Evangelicalism* (IVP, 1976), chapter 5, pp. 87-102.

Robert D. Linder and Richard V. Pierard, *Politics: A Case for Christian Action* (IVP, 1973), chapter 5, pp. 93-120.

Step V

Now write a plan of action as though you were in Joanne's place.

Case Study F:
On Joining a Union

Bill Young was enjoying a great deal of job satisfaction. He had worked as an R.N. for two years in an outstanding burn center. His quest for adventure, excitement and high standards of nursing were all being met. He often flew by helicopter to rescue burn victims, beginning emergency care en route to the hospital. He felt his salary and benefits were more than adequate to support his growing family. As a Christian he felt he could work with freedom and integrity in his present situation. Then the nursing staff voted to unionize. All R.N.'s except those in management positions were required to join the union within two years or find employment elsewhere.

Bill saw the union as a frightening development which he could not join without compromising his Christian values. First of all, he saw no need for the union. Hospital employees were already being treated fairly. The grievances which brought in the union were inherent to nursing and could not really be avoided (for example, working evenings, nights and weekends). Second, if the union were to strike, all members would be forced to join the picket line. Bill had seen what happened at a nearby hospital when nurses went on strike. Those who attempted to cross the picket line were physically attacked. Their car tires were slashed and windshields broken in the parking lot. During the strike patients received minimal care from nursing supervisors, chaplains and interns. Nurses lost a lot more money by being out on strike than they gained by their new contract. Bill did not want to participate in such a strike.

Bill felt that by joining the union he would be endorsing a set of values which were inconsistent with his Christian faith, but if he stayed in his present job he would have no choice. However, he also had deep reservations about resigning. He had a two-year-old son at home, and his wife was six months pregnant. She had just resigned from her job. Nursing positions in the area were scarce, so he might be left with no way to support his family. The trend toward unionization was spreading. He might be faced with the same dilemma all over again if he went to another hospital. ■

The Bible never mentions labor unions per se. Our economic and political systems are very different from anything in the Scriptures. In order to decide whether or not to join a union we need to know more about the union in question, as well as the history of unions in general. What are its goals? Does it use reputable methods? Does it achieve its aims? With the background from study five on economics, justice and social change, we turn now to the Christian's relationship to the world and the family. A decision about whether to join a union must be made in the light of all these considerations.

Steps I—IV.A
Turn to page 99 and answer the questions there in relation to this case study.
Step IV Continued
To complete your evaluation of alternatives answer the questions below, taking into account relevant Scripture and other reading. Remember the Scripture and readings suggested here are not exhaustive. A concordance and Bible dictionary can provide further resources.
The Christian in the World:
1. How is the Christian related to the secular world?

Mt. 5:13-16	Mt. 10:16-20	Mt. 28:19-20
Jn. 17:16-18	2 Cor. 5:20	2 Cor. 6:14-18
1 Thess. 4:9-12		

2. How should we regard our secular work?

Ps. 104:19-23	Mk. 6:3	Lk. 10:7
Lk. 12:16-31	Acts 18:1-4	Eph. 4:28
2 Thess. 3:6-13		

3. What attitudes should characterize the Christian at work?

Mt. 25:14-30	1 Cor. 4:1-2	Gal. 5:1

Gal. 5:13-15   Gal. 5:22-25   Eph. 6:5-9
Col. 3:23
Other Reading:

   John Daniel, *Labor, Industry and the Church* (Concordia, 1957), pp. 113-35.

   Joan London and Henry Anderson, *So Shall Ye Reap* (Thomas Crowell, 1970), pp. 79-98.

   David Lyon, *Christians and Sociology* (IVP, 1975).

   Horst Symanowski, *The Christian Witness in an Industrial Society* (Westminster, 1964), pp. 111-24.

   Gus Tyler, *The Labor Revolution* (Viking, 1967).

Family Responsibilities:

   1. What responsibilities do Christians have toward their families?

Jn. 19:26-27   Eph. 5:21-33   1 Tim. 5:4
1 Tim. 5:8

   2. If acting in accord with Christian principles jeopardizes a person's job and ability to provide for his family, what should he do?

Mt. 6:24-34   Acts 5:27-32   1 Pet. 3:8-17
Other Reading:

   Edith Deen, *Family Living in the Bible* (Pyramid, 1963).

   Michael Green, *New Life, New Lifestyle* (IVP, 1973), pp. 111-19.

   O. R. Johnston, *Who Needs the Family?* (IVP, 1980).

Step V

Now write a plan of action as though you were in Bill's place.

Case Study G:
On Judging Others

It was Alice's first week of work after seven years of "retirement." She felt terribly insecure in the hospital setting, but she had already been put in charge of the thirty-two-bed medical unit. Mrs. Johnson, who had worked at City Hospital for twenty years as an R.N., was on her team. The head nurse had instructed Alice the day before not to assign Mrs. Johnson to give medicines. When Alice asked why, she hedged and said, "Well, she only works part time."

Occasionally patients would complain about Mrs. Johnson, but usually the complaints were nonspecific. Mrs. Johnson would be assigned to other patients the next day and all would be well. Then one day a peculiar thing happened.

Alice was making rounds. When she came to room 602 the door would not open. The patient in room 602, Mr. Kirk, was not able to get out of bed. Alice was concerned that he had tried to get up and perhaps had fallen against the door. Maybe he was unconscious. She called his name. No answer. She called louder, afraid to push the door for fear of injuring Mr. Kirk. Her heart was in her mouth as she shoved the door open a crack to look inside. Furniture tumbled to the floor with a loud crash. Mrs. Johnson stood in the middle of the room with her hands on her hips and shouted, "Can't you respect a person's privacy during his bath?"

Mr. Kirk was sitting naked on a chair, swaying from side to side as he attempted to keep his balance. All the windows were wide open. The room was freezing cold. The bed was stripped and dirty linen was all over the floor. Mr. Kirk looked up, shivering, and said, "I'm so cold, I want to go back to bed."

Alice closed the windows and picked up a sheet, saying, "I'll help you make the bed so Mr. Kirk can get back in it."

Mrs. Johnson was outraged, "He's my patient. I'll do it myself!"

Alice covered Mr. Kirk with a blanket and tried to reassure him, then she made the bed while Mrs. Johnson watched.

Alice was furious. She called Mrs. Johnson out of the room and asked her what she thought she was doing. After she cooled down Alice went to talk to Mr. Kirk. He was smiling, "It feels so good to be back in my bed and warm again," he said. "Please don't send that woman in here again. She's mean!"

After leaving Mr. Kirk's room Alice told Mrs. Johnson that she would care for Mr. Kirk for the rest of the day. When the supervisor made her rounds Alice expressed concern about Mrs. Johnson's strange behavior. The supervisor shared her concern and said, "I wish I knew what we could do about this. It's not the first time she's pulled something like this, but we have to be careful since she's of a minority race."

For the next few weeks Mrs. Johnson seemed to be the ideal nurse. She was gentle and considerate to staff and to patients. Then one day Alice answered a patient's call light. Mrs. Owens, who had severe arthritis in her hands and knees was sitting on the side of her bed, crying into a basin of dirty wash water.

"You seem upset," Alice said as she entered the room.

"My knees hurt so bad!" she responded.

"Did something happen?" Alice asked.

Mrs. Owens sat and cried, biting her lip. She seemed to be wrestling with something inside herself. "That nurse who was helping me with my bath told me to straighten my leg. I couldn't do it. I have arthritis, you know. I tried to tell her, but she just grabbed my leg and pushed my knee down with her hand. It hurts so bad. I told her to get out, but I can't finish my bath sitting here. I can't wring out the washcloth well enough to keep it from dripping over everything. They usually let me sit in the shower, but that nurse told me I couldn't. She said she would wash me."

Alice brought Mrs. Owens some pain medication and went to look for Mrs. Johnson. She was sitting in the nurses' lounge smoking a cigarette.

"What happened with Mrs. Owens?" Alice asked.

"She didn't want my help," Mrs. Johnson replied.

"She claims you pushed her knee straight by force," Alice countered.

"She wasn't moving fast enough. I was just helping her," she replied.

"Then you did do it," Alice responded as Mrs. Johnson nodded in agreement.

"Well, I think we need to fill out an incident report, and I'd like to discuss the matter with the supervisor," Alice replied. Alice's voice trembled as she called the supervisor.

The supervisor came up immediately. First she checked on Mrs. Owens. Then, coming out of the room with tears in her eyes, she said, "Tell Mrs. Johnson that I want to see her in the nursing office in ten minutes. She might as well bring her coat with her."

Later that afternoon the supervisor came back. "We have a dilemma on our hands," she began. "As you know this is not the first incident we've had with Mrs. Johnson. I don't think it is safe to let her continue on our staff. Do you realize how serious a charge that is? If we fire her, she may never be able to get a nursing job again. She has a family to support. She will probably sue the hospital. She may take revenge on you and me and possibly others. The last time we tried to fire a minority member a militant group planted bombs on the porch of the head nurse involved. I'm glad you've been willing to stand up to her behavior. You've presented us with evidence we can't ignore. I'm going to ask you to put yourself on the line some more. Would you be willing to write up every single incident with as much detail as possible? I need it for her file in case she does sue." ■

Most Christians have been raised with the admonition of Matthew 7:1 engraved deeply upon them, "Judge not, that ye be not judged." Judging is God's business, not ours (Jas. 4:11; Rom. 12:19), and we try desperately to refrain from using our critical faculties. But there is another side of the picture. In Luke 12:57 Jesus admonishes the crowd, "And why do you not judge for yourselves what is right?" In John 7:24 Jesus says, "Do not judge by appearances, but judge with right judgment." There is a time and a place to pass judgment. As Christians we have the responsibility to judge fairly and honestly.

Steps I—IV.A
Turn to page 99 and answer the questions there in relation to this case study.

Step IV Continued
To complete your evaluation of alternatives answer the questions below, taking into account relevant Scripture and other reading. Remember the Scripture and readings suggested here are not exhaustive. A concordance and Bible dictionary can provide further resources.

Judging Others:
1. What risk do you take by judging someone?

Mt. 7:1   Rom. 2:1-11

2. What qualifications and limits does Jesus set on your ability to judge?

Mt. 7:2-5   Jn. 8:15-16

3. What attitudes should characterize a Christian's relationships with wrongdoers?

Rom. 12:14-21   Eph. 4:31-32   Gal. 3:12-14

4. What procedure should you follow when you judge someone's behavior to be wrong?

Mt. 18:15-20   1 Tim. 5:20

Other Reading:

John W. Alexander, *Practical Criticism* (IVP, 1976).

David Augsburger, *Caring Enough to Confront* (Regal, 1973).

Step V
Now write a plan of action as though you were in Alice's place.

Case Study H:
On Inflicting
Values on Others

Joe Harper was excited about going to work this morning. The Bible study he attended last night had been on John 14. He could hardly wait to share what he had learned with Mr. Strauss.

Mr. Strauss was dying. He knew he was dying, and he was scared. He had been a fairly religious Jew all his life, but as death approached, God seemed very far away. Joe had seen him reading his prayer book each day and commented to him about it. After that they talked about God almost every time Joe was in Mr. Strauss's room. Mr. Strauss always brought up the subject.

Today Joe started the conversation, "Mr. Strauss, you don't have to be alone when you die! Let me read you something." Joe pulled his New Testament from his uniform pocket and read from John 14, " 'And when I go and prepare a place for you, I will come again and will take you to myself, that where I am you may be also.' Jesus is going to be with you, Mr. Strauss. You have to trust him, though."

"I don't know too much about your Jesus," Mr. Strauss responded. "Tell me some more."

Joe sat down and explained the gospel to Mr. Strauss.

"I believe in Jesus now," Mr. Strauss interjected as Joe talked. "I guess that makes me a Christian." Excitedly Joe prayed with Mr. Strauss as he verbally committed his life to Christ.

Later, Mrs. Strauss visited her husband. Mr. Strauss shared his good news with her. She was indignant. She went to the nursing office and reported Joe for proselytizing. Joe was reprimanded by his supervisor, and a memorandum was sent to all floors stating that hospital personnel would not be permitted to discuss religion or distribute any form of religious literature in the hospital. ■

Evangelism on the job presents Christians with two major temptations. The most prevalent one is to put nursing into a compartment of our lives separate from our faith. Here the Christian may go on evangelistic projects with other Christians, or speak freely to colleagues about Christ, but never mention spiritual concerns with patients. This person may feel that it is unfair to "hit a person with the gospel when they're down." The other extreme is the Christian who goes into every patient's room with a tract or a pat presentation of the gospel. Between these two extremes, is there a legitimate place for evangelism with patients?

Steps I—IV.A

Turn to page 99 and answer the questions there in relation to this case study.

Step IV Continued

To complete your evaluation of alternatives answer the questions below, taking into account relevant Scripture and other reading. Remember the Scripture and readings suggested here are not exhaustive. A concordance and Bible dictionary can provide further resources.

Evangelism on the Job:

1. Is evangelism appropriate in a nursing context? Why or why not?

Job 6:6-13	Is. 53:4-6	Is. 61:1-3
2 Tim. 4:1-5	Jas. 2:14-18	Jas. 5:13-20

2. What relationship did Jesus' healing ministry have to his message?

Mk. 2:1-12	Mk. 10:46-52	Lk. 17:11-19
Jn. 5:2-14		

3. What attitudes and actions should characterize our efforts to share Christ with patients?

2 Cor. 4:1-2	Eph. 5:1-2	Col. 3:12-17
1 Thess. 2:3-8	Tit. 3:8-9	Jas. 3:13-18
1 Pet. 1:21	1 Pet. 3:15-16	

4. What can Christians do if policies are made to prohibit evangelism?

Acts 5:27-29	2 Cor. 4:7-16	2 Cor. 5:11
Col. 4:2-6	Heb. 12:11-15	

Other Reading:

Sharon Fish and Judith Allen Shelly, *Spiritual Care: The Nurse's Role* (IVP, 1978).

Paul E. Little et al., *HIS Guide to Evangelism* (IVP, 1977).

Richard E. Morgan, *The Supreme Court and Religion* (Free Press, 1972).

Rebecca Manley Pippert, *Out of the Saltshaker* (IVP, 1979).

Mary Thompson, *Lifestyle of Love* (IVP, 1978).

Step V

Now write a plan of action as though you were in Joe's place.

Guidelines for Discussion Groups

Session 1: What Is Your Philosophy of Nursing?
Preparation:
1. Complete the preliminary study on "A Christian Philosophy of Nursing," pp. 96-98.
2. Read chapters 1 and 2, and appendix A, "Codes of Ethics."
Discussion:
1. Share and discuss your answers to the questions in the exercise on "A Christian Philosophy of Nursing."
2. Construct a chart summarizing the beliefs expressed in the codes of ethics in appendix A. (Use a chalkboard or overhead projector.)
   a. What does each code say about the role of the nurse (for example, rights, responsibilities, image)?
   b. How are patients viewed in each (rights, responsibilities, image)?
3. Are there statements in any of the codes with which you cannot agree? On what basis?

Session 2: What Do You Believe About the Right to Live/Right to Die?
Preparation:
1. Read chapters 6 and 8, and appendixes B and C.
2. Using guidelines in chapters 6 and 8 do independent biblical studies on life and death.
Discussion:
1. Share your conclusions from studying life and death in Scripture.
2. Evaluate the views of life and death expressed in the different requests for withholding of heroic measures in appendix B. Are these views

compatible with your conclusions from your own biblical research? If not, how do they differ?

3. Summarize the basic statements of the California Natural Death Act. If such a law were on the books in your state, would you sign a "Directive to Physicians" form? For what reasons?

Sessions 3—10: Examining the Issues (Case Studies A—H)
Preparation:

1. Read chapters 1—8.

2. Work through all the steps in the decision-making process for the case study to be discussed.

Discussion:

1. What was your first reaction to the situation?

2. Share your responses to the questions in Step I concerning emotional responses, personal biases, cultural values and communication problems.

3. Share the information you collected in Step II about the issues at stake. Did this added information change your perspective on the situation? How?

4. List some of the alternatives you proposed in Step III.

5. Summarize the biblical insights you gained into the issues at stake. How did what you discovered in the Bible affect your view of the issues?

6. Discuss one or two of the proposed plans of action developed in Step V. What are the pros and cons of each?

7. Share any personal experiences where similar issues were at stake. What did you do? What was the result of your action (or inaction)?

Appendix A:
Codes of Ethics

American Nurses' Association
Code for Nurses

Preamble
The *Code for Nurses* is based on belief about the nature of individuals, nursing, health, and society. Recipients and providers of nursing services are viewed as individuals and groups who possess basic rights and responsibilities, and whose values and circumstances command respect at all times. Nursing encompasses the promotion and restoration of health, the prevention of illness, and the alleviation of suffering. The statements of the *Code* and their interpretation provide guidance for conduct and relationships in carrying out nursing responsibilities consistent with the ethical obligations of the profession and quality in nursing care.

Code for Nurses
1. The nurse provides services with respect for human dignity and the uniqueness of the client unrestricted by considerations of social or economic status, personal attributes, or the nature of health problems.

2. The nurse safeguards the client's right to privacy by judiciously protecting information of a confidential nature.

3. The nurse acts to safeguard the client and the public when health care and safety are affected by the incompetent, unethical, or illegal practice of any person.

4. The nurse assumes responsibility and accountability for individual nursing judgments and actions.

5. The nurse maintains competence in nursing.

6. The nurse exercises informed judgment and uses individual competence and qualifications as criteria in seeking consultation, accepting responsibilities, and delegating nursing activities to others.

7. The nurse participates in activities that contribute to the ongoing development of the profession's body of knowledge.

8. The nurse participates in the profession's efforts to implement and improve standards of nursing.

9. The nurse participates in the profession's efforts to establish and maintain conditions of employment conducive to high quality nursing care.

10. The nurse participates in the profession's effort to protect the public from misinformation and misrepresentation and to maintain the integrity of nursing.

11. The nurse collaborates with members of the health professions and other citizens in promoting community and national efforts to meet the health needs of the public.

International Council of Nurses Code for Nurses Ethical Concepts Applied to Nursing 1973

The fundamental responsibility of the nurse is fourfold: to promote health, to prevent illness, to restore health and to alleviate suffering.

The need for nursing is universal. Inherent in nursing is respect for life, dignity and rights of man. It is unrestricted by considerations of nationality, race, creed, colour, age, sex, politics or social status.

Nurses render health services to the individual, the family and the community and coordinate their services with those of related groups.

Nurses and People

The nurse's primary responsibility is to those people who require nursing care.

The nurse, in providing care, promotes an environment in which the values, customs and spiritual beliefs of the individual are respected.

The nurse holds in confidence personal information and uses judgement in sharing this information.

Nurses and Practice

The nurse carries personal responsibility for nursing practice and for maintaining competence by continual learning.

The nurse maintains the highest standards of nursing care possible within the reality of a specific situation.

The nurse uses judgement in relation to individual competence when accepting and delegating responsibilities.

The nurse when acting in a professional capacity should at all times maintain standards of personal conduct which reflect credit upon the profession.

Nurses and Society

The nurse shares with other citizens the responsibility for initiating and supporting action to meet the health and social needs of the public.

Nurses and Co-Workers

The nurse sustains a cooperative relationship with co-workers in nursing and other fields.

The nurse takes appropriate action to safeguard the individual when his care is endangered by a co-worker or any other person.

Nurses and the Profession

The nurse plays the major role in determining and implementing desirable standards of nursing practice and nursing education.

The nurse is active in developing a core of professional knowledge.

The nurse, acting through the professional organization, participates in establishing and maintaining equitable social and economic working conditions in nursing.

Adopted by the ICN Council of National Representatives, Mexico City in May 1973.

American Hospital Association
A Patient's Bill of Rights

1. The patient has the right to considerate and respectful care.

2. The patient has the right to obtain from his physician complete current information concerning his diagnosis, treatment, and prognosis in terms the patient can be reasonably expected to understand. When it is not medically advisable to give such information to the patient, the information should be made available to an appropriate person in his behalf. He has the right to know by name, the physician responsible for coordinating his care.

3. The patient has the right to receive from his physician information necessary to give informed consent prior to the start of any procedure and/or treatment. Except in emergencies, such information for informed consent should include but not necessarily be limited to the specific procedure and/or treatment, the medically significant risks involved, and the probable duration of incapacitation. Where medically significant alternatives for care or treatment exist, or when the patient requests information concerning medical alternatives, the patient has the right to such information. The patient also has the right to know the name of the person responsible for the procedures and/or treatment.

4. The patient has the right to refuse treatment to the extent permitted by law and to be informed of the medical consequences of his action.

5. The patient has the right to every consideration of his privacy concerning his own medical care program. Case discussion, consultation, examination, and treatment are confidential and should be conducted discreetly. Those not directly involved in his care must have the permission of the patient to be present.

6. The patient has the right to expect that all communications and records pertaining to his care should be treated as confidential.

7. The patient has the right to expect that within its capacity a hospital must make reasonable response to the request of a patient for services. The hospital must provide evaluation, service, and/or referral as indicated by the urgency of the case. When medically permissible a patient may be transferred to another facility only after he has received complete information and explanation concerning the needs for and alternatives to such a transfer. The institution to which the patient is to be transferred must first have accepted the patient for transfer.

8. The patient has the right to obtain information as to any relationship of his hospital to other health care and educational institutions insofar as his care is concerned. The patient has the right to obtain information as to the existence of any professional relationships among individuals, by name, who are treating him.

9. The patient has the right to be advised if the hospital proposes to engage in or perform human experimentation affecting his care or treatment. The patient has the right to refuse to participate in such research projects.

10. The patient has the right to expect reasonable continuity of care. He has the right to know in advance what appointment times and physicians are available and where. The patient has the right to expect that the hospital will provide a mechanism whereby he is informed by his physician or a delegate of the physician of the patient's continuing health care requirements following discharge.

11. The patient has the right to examine and receive an explanation of his bill regardless of source of payment.

12. The patient has the right to know what hospital rules and regulations apply to his conduct as a patient.

Appendix B: Requests to Withhold Heroic Measures

Living Will

To My Family, My Physician, My Lawyer and All Others
Whom It May Concern

Death is as much a reality as birth, growth, maturity and old age—it is the one certainty of life. If the time comes when I can no longer take part in decisions for my own future, let this statement stand as an expression of my wishes and directions, while I am still of sound mind.

If at such a time the situation should arise in which there is no reasonable expectation of my recovery from extreme physical or mental disability, I direct that I be allowed to die and not be kept alive by medications, artificial means or "heroic measures". I do, however, ask that medication be mercifully administered to me to alleviate suffering even though this may shorten my remaining life.

This statement is made after careful consideration and is in accordance with my strong convictions and beliefs. I want the wishes and directions here expressed carried out to the extent permitted by law. Insofar as they are not legally enforceable, I hope that those to whom this Will is addressed will regard themselves as morally bound by these provisions.

Signed_____

Date_____

Witness_____

Witness_____

Copies of this request have been given to _____

Catholic Health Association

Christian Affirmation of Life

To my family, friends, physician, lawyer, and clergyman:

I believe that each individual person is created by God our Father in love and that God retains a loving relationship to each person throughout human life and eternity.

I believe that Jesus Christ lived, suffered, and died for me and that his suffering, death, and resurrection prefigure and make possible the death-resurrection process which I now anticipate.

I believe that each person's worth and dignity derives from the relationship of love in Christ that God has for each individual person and not from one's usefulness or effectiveness in society.

I believe that God our Father has entrusted to me a shared dominion with him over my earthly existence so that I am bound to use ordinary means to preserve my life but I am free to refuse extraordinary means to prolong my life.

I believe that through death life is not taken away but merely changed, and though I may experience fear, suffering, and sorrow, by the grace of the Holy Spirit, I hope to accept death as a free human act which enables me to surrender this life and to be united with God for eternity.

Because of my belief:

I request that I be informed as death approaches so that I may continue to prepare for the full encounter with Christ through the help of the sacraments and the consolation and prayers of my family and friends.

I request that, if possible, I be consulted concerning the medical procedures which might be used to prolong my life as death approaches.

If I can no longer take part in decisions concerning my own future and if there is no reasonable expectation of my recovery from physical and mental disability, I request that no extraordinary means be used to prolong my life.

I request, though I wish to join my suffering to the suffering of Jesus so I may be united fully with him in the act of death—resurrection, that my pain, if unbearable, be alleviated. However, no means should be used with the intention of shortening my life.

I request, because I am a sinner and in need of reconciliation and because my faith, hope, and love may not overcome all fear and doubt, that my family, friends, and the whole Christian community join me in prayer and mortification as I prepare for the great personal act of dying.

Finally, I request that after my death, my family, my friends, and the whole Christian community pray for me, and rejoice with me because of the mercy and love of the Trinity with whom I hope to be united for all eternity.

signed _____ date _____

American Protestant Hospital Association

A Personal Statement of Faith

I believe that every person is created by God as an individual of value and dignity. My basic worth and value as a person is inherent in the relationship of love that God has for me and not in my usefulness in society.

I believe that God has endowed me as His creature with the responsibility and privilege of sharing with God in the dominion over my earthly existence. I believe in the sanctity of human life which is to be celebrated in the spirit of creative living because it does have worth, meaning, and purpose. Therefore, I am responsible to use all ordinary means to preserve my life.

I further believe, however, that every human life is given dignity in dying, as well as in living. Therefore, I am free to refuse artificial and heroic measures to prolong my dying. I affirm my human right which allows me to die my own death within the limits of social, legal and spiritual factors.

I believe I have the right to die with dignity—respected, cared for, loved and inspired by hope. I consider as unjust the continuation of artificial and mechanical life support systems through expensive medical and technological means when there is no reasonable expectation for my recovery of meaningful personal life.

In order to avoid the useless prolongation of my dying and the suffering of my loved ones, I am signing a document making known my will regarding my medical treatment in the case of my terminal illness.

Instructions for My Care in the Event of Terminal Illness

My faith affirms that life is a gift of God and that physical death is a part of life and is the completed stage of a person's development. My faith assures me that even in death there is hope and the sustaining grace and love of God. Because of my belief, I wish this statement to stand as the testament of my wishes.

I, _____, request that I be fully informed as my death approaches. If possible, I want to participate in decisions regarding my medical treatment and the procedures which may be used to prolong my life. If there is no reasonable expectation of my recovery from physical or mental disability, I direct my physician and all medical personnel not to prolong my life by artificial or mechanical means. I direct that I receive pain and symptom control. However, this decision is not a request that direct intervention be taken to shorten my life.

This decision is made after careful consideration and reflection. I direct that all legal means be taken to support my choice. In the carrying out of my will as stated, I release all physicians and other health personnel, all institutions and their employees and members of my family from legal culpability and responsibility.

Signed_____

Date _____

Witnessed By: _____

_____

Appendix C: California Natural Death Act

California Natural Death Act

Assembly Bill No. 3060
Chapter 1439
An act to add Chapter 3.9 (commencing with Section 7185) to Part 1
of Division 7 of the Health and Safety Code, relating to medical care.

*[Approved by Governor September 30, 1976. Filed with Secretary of
State September 30, 1976.]*

Legislative Counsel's Digest
AB 3060, Keene. Cessation of medical care for terminal patients.

No existing statute prescribes a procedure whereby a person may
provide in advance for the withholding or withdrawal of medical care in
the event the person should suffer a terminal illness or mortal injury.

This bill would expressly authorize the withholding or withdrawal of
life-sustaining procedures, as defined, from adult patients afflicted with a
terminal condition, as defined, where the patient has executed a directive
in the form and manner prescribed by the bill. Such a directive would
generally be effective for 5 years from the date of execution unless sooner
revoked in a specified manner. This bill would relieve physicians,
licensed health professionals acting under the direction of a physician,
and health facilities from civil liability, and would relieve physicians and
licensed health professionals acting under the direction of a physician
from criminal prosecution or charges of unprofessional conduct, for withholding or withdrawing life-sustaining procedures in accordance with
the provisions of the bill.

The bill would provide that such a withholding or withdrawal of life-sustaining procedures shall not constitute a suicide nor impair or invalidate life insurance, and the bill would specify that the making of such a directive shall not restrict, inhibit, or impair the sale, procurement, or issuance of life insurance or modify existing life insurance. The bill would provide that health insurance carriers, as prescribed, could not require execution of a directive as a condition for being insured for, or receiving, health care services.

The bill would make it a misdemeanor to willfully conceal, cancel, deface, obliterate, or damage the directive of another without the declarant's consent. Any person, not justified or excused by law, who falsifies or forges the directive of another or willfully conceals or withholds personal knowledge of a prescribed revocation with the intent to cause a withholding or withdrawal of life-sustaining procedures contrary to the wishes of the declarant and thereby causes life-sustaining procedures to be withheld or withdrawn, and death to thereby be hastened, would be subject to prosecution for unlawful homicide.

This bill would also provide that, notwithstanding Section 2231 of the Revenue and Taxation Code, there shall be no reimbursement nor appropriation made by this bill for a specified reason.

The people of the State of California do enact as follows:

Section 1.   Chapter 3.9 (commencing with Section 7185) is added to Part 1 of Division 7 of the Health and Safety Code, to read:

Chapter 3.9. Natural Death Act

7185.   This act shall be known and may be cited as the Natural Death Act.

7186.   The Legislature finds that adult persons have the fundamental right to control the decisions relating to the rendering of their own medical care, including the decision to have life-sustaining procedures withheld or withdrawn in instances of a terminal condition.

The Legislature further finds that modern medical technology has made possible the artificial prolongation of human life beyond natural limits.

The Legislature further finds that, in the interest of protecting individual autonomy, such prolongation of life for persons with a terminal condition may cause loss of patient dignity and unnecessary pain and suffering, while providing nothing medically necessary or beneficial to the patient.

The Legislature further finds that there exists considerable uncertainty in the medical and legal professions as to the legality of terminating the use or application of life-sustaining procedures where the patient has voluntarily and in sound mind evidenced a desire that such procedures be withheld or withdrawn.

In recognition of the dignity and privacy which patients have a right to expect, the Legislature hereby declares that the laws of the State of California shall recognize the right of an adult person to make a written directive instructing his physician to withhold or withdraw life-sustaining procedures in the event of a terminal condition.

7187. The following definitions shall govern the construction of this chapter:

(a) "Attending physician" means the physician selected by, or assigned to, the patient who has primary responsibility for the treatment and care of the patient.

(b) "Directive" means a written document voluntarily executed by the declarant in accordance with the requirements of Section 7188. The directive, or a copy of the directive, shall be made part of the patient's medical records.

(c) "Life-sustaining procedure" means any medical procedure or intervention which utilizes mechanical or other artificial means to sustain, restore, or supplant a vital function, which, when applied to a qualified patient, would serve only to artifically prolong the moment of death and where, in the judgment of the attending physician, death is imminent whether or not such procedures are utilized. "Life-sustaining procedure" shall not include the administration of medication or the performance of any medical procedure deemed necessary to alleviate pain.

(d) "Physician" means a physician and surgeon licensed by the Board of Medical Quality Assurance or the Board of Osteopathic Examiners.

(e) "Qualified patient" means a patient diagnosed and certified in writing to be afflicted with a terminal condition by two physicians, one of whom shall be the attending physician, who have personally examined the patient.

(f) "Terminal condition" means an incurable condition caused by injury, disease, or illness, which, regardless of the application of life-sustaining procedures, would, within reasonable medical judgment, produce death, and where the application of life-sustaining procedures serve only to postpone the moment of death of the patient.

7188.   Any adult person may execute a directive directing the withholding or withdrawal of life-sustaining procedures in a terminal condition. The directive shall be signed by the declarant in the presence of two witnesses not related to the declarant by blood or marriage and who would not be entitled to any portion of the estate of the declarant upon his decease under any will of the declarant or codicil thereto then existing or, at the time of the directive, by operation of law then existing. In addition, a witness to a directive shall not be the attending physician, an employee of the attending physician or a health facility in which the declarant is a patient, or any person who has a claim against any portion of the estate of the declarant upon his decease at the time of the execution of the directive. The directive shall be in the following form:

Directive to Physicians

Directive made this _____ day of _____ (month, year).

I _____, being of sound mind, willfully, and voluntarily make known my desire that my life shall not be artificially prolonged under the circumstances set forth below, do hereby declare:

1. If at any time I should have an incurable injury, disease, or illness certified to be a terminal condition by two physicians, and where the application of life-sustaining procedures would serve only to artificially prolong the moment of my death and where my physician determines that my death is imminent whether or not life-sustaining procedures are utilized, I direct that such procedures be withheld or withdrawn, and that I be permitted to die naturally.

2. In the absence of my ability to give directions regarding the use of such life-sustaining procedures, it is my intention that this directive shall be honored by my family and physician(s) as the final expression of my legal right to refuse medical or surgical treatment and accept the consequences from such refusal.

3. If I have been diagnosed as pregnant and that diagnosis is known to my physician, this directive shall have no force or effect during the course of my pregnancy.

4. I have been diagnosed and notified at least 14 days ago as having a terminal condition by _____, M.D., whose address is _____ and whose telephone number is _____. I understand that if I have not filled in the physician's name and address, it shall be presumed that I did not have a terminal condition when I made out this directive.

5. This directive shall have no force or effect five years from the date filled in above.

6. I understand the full import of this directive and I am emotionally and mentally competent to make this directive.

Signed _____

City, County and State of Residence _____

The declarant has been personally known to me and I believe him or her to be of sound mind.

Witness _____

Witness _____

7188.5.   A directive shall have no force or effect if the declarant is a patient in a skilled nursing facility as defined in subdivision (c) of Section 1250 at the time the directive is executed unless one of the two witnesses to the directive is a patient advocate or ombudsman as may be designated by the State Department of Aging for this purpose pursuant to any other applicable provision of law. The patient advocate or ombudsman shall have the same qualifications as a witness under Section 7188.

The intent of this section is to recognize that some patients in skilled nursing facilities may be so insulated from a voluntary decisionmaking role, by virtue of the custodial nature of their care, as to require special assurance that they are capable of willfully and voluntarily executing a directive.

7189.   (a) A directive may be revoked at any time by the declarant, without regard to his mental state or competency, by any of the following methods:

(1) By being canceled, defaced, obliterated, or burnt, torn, or otherwise destroyed by the declarant or by some person in his presence and by his direction.

(2) By a written revocation of the declarant expressing his intent to revoke, signed and dated by the declarant. Such revocation shall become effective only upon communication to the attending physician by

the declarant or by a person acting on behalf of the declarant. The attending physician shall record in the patient's medical record the time and date when he received notification of the written revocation.

(3) By a verbal expression by the declarant of his intent to revoke the directive. Such revocation shall become effective only upon communication to the attending physician by the declarant or by a person acting on behalf of the declarant. The attending physician shall record in the patient's medical record the time, date, and place of the revocation and the time, date, and place, if different, of when he received notification of the revocation.

(b) There shall be no criminal or civil liability on the part of any person for failure to act upon a revocation made pursuant to this section unless that person has actual knowledge of the revocation.

7189.5.   A directive shall be effective for five years from the date of execution thereof unless sooner revoked in a manner prescribed in Section 7189. Nothing in this chapter shall be construed to prevent a declarant from reexecuting a directive at any time in accordance with the formalities of Section 7188, including reexecution subsequent to a diagnosis of a terminal condition. If the declarant has executed more than one directive, such time shall be determined from the date of execution of the last directive known to the attending physician. If the declarant becomes comatose or is rendered incapable of communicating with the attending physician, the directive shall remain in effect for the duration of the comatose condition or until such time as the declarant's condition renders him or her able to communicate with the attending physician.

7190.   No physician or health facility which, acting in accordance with the requirements of this chapter, causes the withholding or withdrawal of life-sustaining procedures from a qualified patient, shall be subject to civil liability therefrom. No licensed health professional, acting under the direction of a physician, who participates in the withholding or withdrawal of life-sustaining procedures in accordance with the provisions of this chapter shall be subject to any civil liability. No physician, or licensed health professional acting under the direction of a physician, who participates in the withholding or withdrawal of life-sustaining procedures in accordance with the provisions of this chapter shall be guilty of any criminal act or of unprofessional conduct.

7191. (a) Prior to effecting a withholding or withdrawal of life-sustaining procedures from a qualified patient pursuant to the directive, the attending physician shall determine that the directive complies with Section 7188, and, if the patient is mentally competent, that the directive and all steps proposed by the attending physician to be undertaken are in accord with the desires of the qualified patient.

(b) If the declarant was a qualified patient at least 14 days prior to executing or reexecuting the directive, the directive shall be conclusively presumed, unless revoked, to be the directions of the patient regarding the withholding or withdrawal of life-sustaining procedures. No physician, and no licensed health professional acting under the direction of a physician, shall be criminally or civilly liable for failing to effectuate the directive of the qualified patient pursuant to this subdivision. A failure by a physician to effectuate the directive of a qualified patient pursuant to this division shall constitute unprofessional conduct if the physician refuses to make the necessary arrangements, or fails to take the necessary steps, to effect the transfer of the qualified patient to another physician who will effectuate the directive of the qualified patient.

(c) If the declarant becomes a qualified patient subsequent to executing the directive, and has not subsequently reexecuted the directive, the attending physician may give weight to the directive as evidence of the patient's directions regarding the withholding or withdrawal of life-sustaining procedures and may consider other factors, such as information from the affected family or the nature of the patient's illness, injury, or disease, in determining whether the totality of circumstances known to the attending physician justify effectuating the directive. No physician, and no licensed health professional acting under the direction of a physician, shall be criminally or civilly liable for failing to effectuate the directive of the qualified patient pursuant to this subdivision.

7192. (a) The withholding or withdrawal of life-sustaining procedures from a qualified patient in accordance with the provisions of this chapter shall not, for any purpose, constitute a suicide.

(b) The making of a directive pursuant to Section 7188 shall not restrict, inhibit, or impair in any manner the sale, procurement, or issuance of any policy of life insurance, nor shall it be deemed to modify the terms of an existing policy of life insurance. No policy of life insurance shall be legally impaired or invalidated in any manner by the withholding or withdrawal of life-sustaining procedures from an insured qualified patient, notwithstanding any term of the policy to the contrary.

(c) No physician, health facility, or other health provider, and no health care service plan, insurer issuing disability insurance, self-insured employee welfare benefit plan, or nonprofit hospital service plan, shall require any person to execute a directive as a condition for being insured for, or receiving, health care services.

7193. Nothing in this chapter shall impair or supersede any legal right or legal responsibility which any person may have to effect the withholding or withdrawal of life-sustaining procedures in any lawful manner. In such respect the provisions of this chapter are cumulative.

7194. Any person who willfully conceals, cancels, defaces, obliterates, or damages the directive of another without such declarant's consent shall be guilty of a misdemeanor. Any person who, except where justified or excused by law, falsifies or forges the directive of another, or willfully conceals or withholds personal knowledge of a revocation as provided in Section 7189, with the intent to cause a withholding or withdrawal of life-sustaining procedures contrary to the wishes of the declarant, and thereby, because of any such act, directly causes life-sustaining procedures to be withheld or withdrawn and death to thereby be hastened, shall be subject to prosecution for unlawful homicide as provided in Chapter 1 (commencing with Section 187) of Title 8 of Part 1 of the Penal Code.

7195. Nothing in this chapter shall be construed to condone, authorize, or approve mercy killing, or to permit any affirmative or deliberate act or omission to end life other than to permit the natural process of dying as provided in this chapter.

Sec. 2. If any provision of this act or the application thereof to any person or circumstances is held invalid, such invalidity shall not affect other provisions or applications of the act which can be given effect without the invalid provision or application, and to this end the provisions of this act are severable.

Sec. 3. Notwithstanding Section 2231 of the Revenue and Taxation Code, there shall be no reimbursement pursuant to this section nor shall there be any appropriation made by this act because the Legislature recognizes that during any legislative session a variety of changes to laws relating to crimes and infractions may cause both increased and decreased costs to local government entities and school districts which, in the aggregate, do not result in significant identifiable cost changes.

Notes

Chapter 1
[1]Patrick Romanell, "Ethics, Moral Conflicts, and Choice," *American Journal of Nursing*, (1977), 850.
[2]Myra E. Levine, "Nursing Ethics and the Ethical Nurse," *American Journal of Nursing*, (1977), 845.
[3]Diane Uustal, "Searching for Values," *Sigma Theta Tau/Image*, 9, No. 1 (1977), 15.
[4]Ibid.

Chapter 2
[1]Andrew Jameton, "The Nurse: When Roles and Rules Conflict," *Hastings Center Report*, August 1977, p. 22.
[2]Donald C. Drake, "One Must Die So the Other Might Live," *Nursing Forum*, No. 3-4 (1977), 229.
[3]Leah Curtin, "A Tentative Exploration of Nursing Involvement," *Update on Ethics*, 1, No. 1 (1977), 11.
[4]Ibid., p. 13.
[5]Charlotte A. Aikens, R.N., *Studies in Ethics for Nurses* (Philadelphia: W. B. Sauders Company, 1924), pp. 18-19.
[6]Mila Ann Aroskar, "Ethics in the Nursing Curriculum," *Nursing Outlook*, 25, No. 4 (1977), 260-64; and "Nursing Ethics, The Admirable Standards of Nurses: A Survey Report," *Nursing '74*, September 1974, p. 35.

Chapter 4
[1]Carol Ren Kneisl, "Thoughtful Care for the Dying," *American Journal of Nursing*, (1968), 550-53.
[2]Paul Langham, "Open Forum: On Teaching Ethics to Nurses," *Nursing Forum*, No. 3, 4 (1977), 221.
[3]Rosalee C. Yeaworth, "The Agonizing Decisions in Mental Retardation," *American Journal of Nursing*, (1977), 865

Chapter 6
[1]Bockmuehl, Klaus, "Law and the Spirit: Situation Ethics With a Difference," *Christianity Today*, Feb. 24, 1978, p. 49.
[2]R. Alan Cole, *Exodus* (Downers Grove, Ill.: InterVarsity Press, 1973), p. 177.
[3]Noonan, John T. *The Morality of Abortion* (Cambridge: Harvard Univ. Press, 1970), pp. 3-4.

[4]*Didache,* II: 2.
[5]*Epistle of Barnabas* 19:5.
[6]Noonan, p. 12.

Chapter 8

[1]See Margaret Mead, "The Right to Die," *Nursing Outlook,* 16 (Oct. 1968), 22-25; Joseph Fletcher, *Morals and Medicine* (Boston: Beacon Press, 1954), pp. 172-210; and Michele Anne Cawley, "Euthanasia: Should it be a Choice?" *American Journal of Nursing,* (1977), 859-61.

[2]For example, Yeaworth suggests that amniocentesis and abortion might be required of women carrying a fetus with Down's syndrome since the $900,000 spared for each averted case of severe retardation could then be used to provide "good health care to all" (p. 865).

[3]C. Everett Koop, M.D., *The Right to Live; The Right to Die* (Wheaton, Ill.: Tyndale, 1976), p. 90.

[4]Harley S. Smyth, "Motive and Meaning in Medical Morals," text of speech given at Alliance for Life annual banquet, June 26, 1976.

[5]For example, Roy J. Enquist and Henry L. Wildberger, *Christian Faith and the Dying Patient* (New York: Board of Social Ministry/Lutheran Church in America, 1967); Edwin and Helen Alderfer, ed., *Life and Values* (Scottdale, Pa.: Mennonite Publishing House, 1974); and Donald G. McCarthy, "Euthanasia: Meaning and Challenge," in *Ethical Issues in Nursing* (St. Louis: Catholic Hospital Association, 1976).

[6]Joseph Fletcher, *Morals and Medicine* (Boston: Beacon Press, 1954), pp. 172-210.
[7]Ibid., p. 208.
[8]Helmut Thielicke, *The Doctor as Judge of Who Shall Live and Who Shall Die* (Philadelphia: Fortress, 1976), p. 17.
[9]Leah Curtin, *The Mask of Euthanasia* (published by author, 1975, 1976), p. 35.
[10]Francis Schaeffer, *The Mark of the Christian* (Downers Grove, Ill.: InterVarsity Press, 1970).
[11]Augsburger, David, *Caring Enough to Confront* (Glendale, Cal.: Regal, 1973).
[12]Dosia Carlson, *The Unbroken Vigil* (Richmond: John Knox, 1968).

An Annotated Bibliography for Nursing Ethics

I. General Ethics:
A. Books:

Birch, Bruce, and Rasmussen, Larry. *Bible and Ethics in the Christian Life*. Minneapolis, Minn.: Augsburg, 1976. A helpful book for basic understanding in ethics which discusses how to relate Scripture and ethics.

Bonhoeffer, Dietrich. *Ethics*. New York: Macmillan, 1949. A philosophical presentation on ethics in the Christian life. Includes helpful discussion on how the effects of the Fall complicate making moral decisions.

Brunner, Emil. *The Divine Imperative*. Philadelphia: Westminster, 1937. A treatment of human freedom and responsibility.

Buber, Martin. *I and Thou*. Trans. Walter Kaufman. New York: Charles Scribner's Sons, 1970. A philosophical exploration of I-Thou relationship by a Hasidic Jew.

Duska, Ronald, and Whelan, Mariellen. *Moral Development—A Guide to Piaget and Kohlberg*. New York: Paulist Press, 1975. Summarizes stages and phases of moral development described by psychologists Piaget and Kohlberg. Helpful for understanding behavior and basis for ethical decisions as well as assisting people to mature in ethical decision making. Includes a chapter relating the concepts to Christianity.

Fagothey, Austin. *Right and Reason*. 5th ed. St. Louis: C. V. Mosby, 1972. Deals with elements of ethical theory and practice from a Thomistic point of view.

Field, David. *Free to Do Right*. Downers Grove, Ill.: IVP, 1975. The author discusses frequent dilemmas in personal ethics and provides help for those staggered by moral choice.

Field, David. *Taking Sides*. Downers Grove, Ill.: IVP, 1976. The author presents a biblical approach to the knottiest problems facing society: ecology, abortion, divorce, work in an industrial society and race.

Haring, Bernard. *Medical Ethics*. Notre Dame, Ind.: Fides Publishers, 1973. A Catholic theologian discusses implications for medicine of the following questions: What is the nature of man, human life, death, human health?

Hatfield, Charles, ed. *The Scientist and Ethical Decisions*. Downers Grove, Ill.: IVP, 1973. Fourteen Christian scholars grapple with the ethical dilemmas confronting modern scientists. Articles attempt to face dilemmas with the assumption that human values must control human technology.

Hunt, John. *Ethics in a Medical Context.* Palo Alto, Cal.: Mayflower, 1977.

Kierkegaard, Søren. *Either/Or.* Vol. I Trans. Swenson and Swenson. Vol. II Trans. Walter Lowrie. Princeton: Princeton Univ. Press, 1959. A philosophical differentiation between the aesthetic person and the ethical person.

Kierkegaard, Søren. *Fear and Trembling* and *The Sickness Unto Death.* Trans. by Walter Lowrie. Princeton: Princeton Univ. Press, 1954. A philosophical examination of what constitutes a religious person and what it means to be a person before God.

Lange, Ernst. *Ten Great Freedoms.* Trans. David Priestley. Downers Grove, Ill.: IVP, 1970. The liberation that results through God's graciousness is unfolded in this strikingly illustrated poetic meditation on the Ten Commandments.

Nelson, James. *Human Medicine.* Minneapolis, Minn.: Augsburg, 1973. Thought-provoking, comprehensive coverage of issues.

Nelson, James. *Rediscovering the Person in Medical Care.* Minneapolis, Minn.: Augsburg, 1976. Discusses history and issues in biomedical debates as well as personal needs and rights of patients and families.

Niebuhr, H. Richard. *Christ and Culture.* New York: Harper and Row, 1951.

Niebuhr, H. Richard, and Beach, Waldo. *Christian Ethics.* New York: Ronald Press, 1973. Reviews contributions of Scripture and Christian leaders in history to ethical thought and practice. Surveys current trends and relates them to the main lines of earlier movements.

Niebuhr, Reinhold, *Moral Man and Immoral Society.* New York: Charles Scribner's Sons, 1932.

Niebuhr, Reinhold. *The Nature and Destiny of Man.* Vol. I: "Human Nature." Vol. II: "Human Destiny." New York: Charles Scribner's Sons, 1964.

Oden, Thomas. *Should Treatment Be Terminated?* New York: Harper and Row, 1976. Includes analysis of patient and family rights in issues related to euthanasia, quality vs. sanctity of life, the living will. Gives helpful guidelines in dealing with the issues from a Christian viewpoint.

Ramsey, Paul. *The Patient As Person.* New Haven: Yale, 1970. A Christian perspective on informed consent, death and dying, giving of vital organs, transplants and distribution of limited resources.

Thielicke, Helmut. *The Doctor as Judge of Who Shall Live and Who Shall Die.* Philadelphia: Fortress, 1976. Argues medical progress is not always positive but ambiguous. The issues of forced prolongation of life, being the judge over life and death, PKU mental disease, organ transplants raise central questions concerning nature, destiny and dignity of human existence.

Thielicke, Helmut. *Theological Ethics Vol. I: Foundations.* Philadelphia: Fortress, 1969. A thoroughgoing treatise on ethics from an orthodox Christian view.

Uustal, Diane B. *Values and Ethics: Considerations in Nursing Practice.* South Deerfield, Mass.: Published by author, 1978.

Van Til, Cornelius. *Christian Theistic Ethics.* Philadelphia: den Dulk Christian Foundation, 1971. Conservative theoretical treatment of Christian ethics.

Vaux, Kenneth. *Biomedical Ethics.* Harper and Row: New York, 1974. A concise summary of the historical-cultural positions on medical ethics. Includes a Christian approach to making ethical decisions. Excellent general coverage of the field of ethics.

Wertz, Richard, ed. *Readings on Ethical and Social Issues in Biomedicine.* Englewood, N. J.: Prentice-Hall, 1973. An anthology discussing issues in medicine: human experimentation, biological engineering, transplants, behavior control, mental illness, women and medicine, health-care delivery.

Williams, Preston, ed. *Ethical Issues in Biology and Medicine.* Cambridge, Mass.: Schenkman, 1973. Proceedings of a symposium on the identity and dignity of man.

B. Articles:

Allen, Moyra, R.N., Ph.D. "Ethics of Nursing Practice." *The Canadian Nurse,* Feb. 1974. An analysis of ethical problems reported by Canadian nurses.

Crouch, Muriel. "A Basis for Medical Ethics." Christian Medical Society pamphlet. Discusses Christian principles underlying medical ethics in the past and the need to rethink them in view of clinical practice today.

Denison, John M., M.D. "Which Brothers Do We Keep?" *The Canadian Nurse,* May 1972. Argues that our ethical responsibility in health care extends to all socioeconomic levels of society.

Rabb, J. Douglas. "Implications of Moral and Ethical Issues for Nurses." *Nursing Forum,* 15, No. 2 (1976). Introduces basic information on which to base moral decisions.

II. Ethics in Life and Death Matters:

A. Books:

Anderson, Norman. *Issues of Life & Death.* Downers Grove, Ill.: IVP, 1976. A Christian view of abortion, euthanasia, genetic engineering and birth control.

Bayly, Joseph. *The View from a Hearse.* Elgin, Ill.: David C. Cook, 1969. A Christian view of death from the perspective of a father who has lost three sons.

Bermosk, Loretta S. and Corsini, Raymond J., eds. *Critical Incidents in Nursing.* Philadelphia: Saunders, 1973. Focuses on current controversial issues found in nursing case studies.

Carlozzi, Carl G. *Death and Contemporary Man—The Crisis of Terminal Illness.* Grand Rapids: Eerdmans, 1968. A Christian view of ministering in terminal illness.

Creighton, Helen. *Laws Every Nurse Should Know.* 3rd ed. Philadelphia: Saunders, 1975. Handbook of basic facts of the laws related to nursing. Thorough.

Dealing With Death and Dying. Nursing Skillbook. Horsham, Pa.: InterMed Communications, 1976. An amalgam of views dealing with the nurse's role.

Ethical Issues in Nursing. St. Louis, Mo.: The Catholic Hospital Association, 1976. Contains papers presented at four institutes on Ethical Issues in Nursing given by CHA and the Catholic University of America in 1975-1976.

Koop, C. Everett, M.D. *The Right to Live; The Right to Die.* Wheaton, Ill.: Tyndale, 1976. Written by a Christian pediatric surgeon who presents his own views on abortion and mercy killing.

Lawlserton, Richard. *Care of the Dying.* London: Priory, 1973. Hospice philosophy of care. Includes much information about pain control, symptom control and spiritual support.

Lyons, Catherine. *Organ Transplants: The Moral Issues.* Philadelphia: 1970. A beginning discussion on moral considerations related to prolongation of life, organ transplantation, redefining death.

Wycross, R. G. *The Dying Patient.* Christian Medical Society. Helpful insights and practical ideas for care of the dying. A Christian view of the emphasis and explanation of the hospice concept.

B. Articles:

Beauchamp, J. "Euthanasia and the Nurse Practitioner." *Nursing Digest,* Winter 1976. Emphasizes need to be aware of legal, ethical and medical perspectives of death and euthanasia.

"California Natural Death Act; Guidelines and Directives." *California Hospital Association,* Dec. 22, 1976.

Fletcher, Joseph. "Ethics and Euthanasia." *American Journal of Nursing,* April 1973. Gives moral defense for active euthanasia on the basis of a personalistic code of ethics.

Montgomery, John W. "Do We Have the Right to Die?" *Christianity Today,* Jan. 21, 1977. Reacts to the California Right To Die law.

Rachels, James. "Active and Passive Euthanasia." *Nursing Digest,* Fall 1976. Supports active euthanasia when the decision is made not to prolong life. Charlotte Epstein in "Nursing Implications" responds.

Stuart, Douglas K. "Mercy Killing—Is It Biblical?" *Christianity Today,* Feb. 27, 1976. Discusses implications of one recorded incident in the Bible of active euthanasia, then discusses how Jesus never practiced or championed euthanasia. Encourages a look instead either at healing or benefits of suffering as an alternative.

Weber, Leonard J. "Ethics and Euthanasia." *American Journal of Nursing,* July 1973. Defends the position that "letting the patient go" is ethically acceptable while direct killing is not.

C. Tape:

Gustafson, James. "The Prolongation of Life," Feb. 6, 1975. Available from Fuller Seminary Bookstore, Pasadena, Cal. Discusses from a biblical perspective, changing conditions in society which have brought us to question prolonging life.

III. Ethics: Perspectives on the Beginnings of Life:

A. Books:

Bajema, Clifford. *Abortion and the Meaning of Personhood.* Grand Rapids: Baker, 1974. Considers logically and biblically the question of when life begins.

Gardner, R. F. R. *Abortion: The Personal Dilemma.* Old Tappan, New Jersey: Spire Books, 1974. A Christian gynecologist examines the medical, social and spiritual aspects of abortion.

Shoemaker, Donald. *Abortion, The Bible and The Christian.* Cincinnati:, Hayes Publishing Co., Inc., 1976. Presents a strong, biblical case regarding abortion.

Spitzer, Walter, and Saylor, Carlyle, eds. *Birth Control and the Christian.* Wheaton, Ill.: Tyndale, 1969. Christian Medical Society members establish moral guidelines for birth control which will be medically sound, rooted in a biblical ethic.

Thielicke, Helmut. *The Ethics of Sex.* Grand Rapids: Baker, 1976. Discusses many aspects of sexual life including love, marriage, divorce, birth control and abortion.

Trobisch, Walter. *A Baby Just Now?* Rev. ed. Downers Grove, Ill.: IVP, 1980. Previously published as *Please Help Me! Please Love Me!* Shows importance of both husband and wife seeking God's will together for family planning and marital happiness.

Weber, Leonard, *Who Shall Live?* New York: Paulist Press, 1976. A Catholic exploration of the ethical questions surrounding severe birth defects.

Wilke, Dr. and Mrs. J. C. *Handbook on Abortion.* Cincinnati: Hiltz Publishing Co., 1971. Presents the "Right to Life" or "Pro-Life" view on abortion.

B. Articles:

Cornish, Joan. "Women's Experiences with Abortion," *Current Practice in Obstetric and*

Gynecologic Nursing. Mosby's Current Practice and Perspectives in Nursing series, Vol. I.

Cottrell, Jack. "Abortion and the Mosaic Law." *Christianity Today,* March 16, 1973.

Lanahan, Colleen. "Anxieties and Fears of Patients Seeking Abortion." *Current Practice in Obstetric and Gynecologic Nursing.* Mosby's Current Practice and Perspectives in Nursing series, Vol. I.

Scott, Graham A. D. "Abortion and the Incarnation." *Journal of the Evangelical Theological Society,* Winter 1974.

Smedes, Lewis. "The Abortion Epidemic." *Reformed Journal,* March 1975. Discusses implications of abortion for comfort and convenience of potential parents. Calls for the Christian community to affirm deep respect for human life.

Stott, John R. W. "Reverence for Human Life." *Christianity Today,* June 9, 1972.

IV. Ethics Relating to Patients' Rights:
A. Books:

Annas, George. *The Rights of Hospital Patients.* New York: Avon, 1975. Discusses what patients' rights are from admission to discharge especially for women, children, terminally ill. Considers patients' informed consents, hospital bill payments. Does not discuss ethical issues specifically. Prepared by the American Civil Liberties Union.

B. Articles:

Ashworth, Patricia. "Ethics in the Intensive Care Therapy Unit." *Nursing Mirror and Midwives Journal,* 139, No. 20. Examines dilemmas that ICU nurses face, stressing the importance of nurses' ethical responsibilities.

Bok, Sissela. "The Ethics of Giving Placebos." *Scientific American,* 231, No. 5. Although not dealing with nursing directly, presents good information and facts about placebos and the dangers of deception.

Bush, Patricia. "The Placebo Effect." *Nursing Digest,* Fall 1976. With accompanying article, "Nursing Implications," by Josephine G. Paterson, stimulates individual evaluation responses and value systems in relationship to placebo effects in patient care.

Johnson, Priscilla. "The Long, Hard Dying of Joe Rodriguez." *American Journal of Nursing,* January 1977. Case study of a dying patient and the dilemma that a young nurse faces.

Norton, Doreen. "The Research Ethic." *Nursing Times,* 71, No. 50. Focuses on the problems of nursing research and the responsibility of doing research.

(This bibliography is adapted from one produced by NCF West Coast staff.)